SIMPLE SECRETS

FOR BECOMING

HEALTHY,
WEALTHY,
& WISE

Also in this series

SIMPLE SECRETS

FOR BECOMING

HEALTHY,
WEALTHY,
& WISE

WHAT SCIENTISTS HAVE LEARNED
AND HOW YOU CAN USE IT

DAVID NIVEN, Ph.D.

HarperSanFrancisco
A Division of HarperCollinsPublishers

HarperCollins books may be purchased for educational, business, or sales promotional use. For information please write: Special Markets Department, HarperCollins Publishers, 10 East 53rd Street, New York, NY 10022.

HarperCollins Web site: http://www.harpercollins.com

HarperCollins®, 🏠®, and HarperSanFrancisco™
are trademarks of HarperCollins Publishers.

FIRST EDITION

Library of Congress Cataloging-in-Publication Data
Niven, David.
Simple secrets for becoming healthy, wealthy, and wise : what scientists
have learned and how you can use it / David Niven. — 1st ed.
p. cm.
Includes bibliographical references.
ISBN-10: 0-06-085881-8
ISBN-13: 978-0-06-085881-0
1. Success. 2. Conduct of life. I. Title.
BJ1611.2.N58   2006
158—dc22   2006041200

07 08 09 10 RRD (H) 10 9 8 7 6 5 4 3 2

TO

Patti,

George,

Eileen,

and John

Contents

A Note to Readers

EACH DAY'S ENTRY is based on the research conclusions of scientists studying the topic. Each entry contains a key research finding complemented by advice and an example illustrating the idea. The research conclusions on happiness, success, and relationships are based on meta-analyses of research on those topics, which means that each conclusion is derived from the work of multiple researchers studying the same topic. To enable the reader to find further information on each topic, a reference to a supporting study is included at the end of each entry. Entries on health topics are based solely on the study cited.

This Year's Journey

ONE OF THE greatest teachers I've ever known talked endlessly about the concept of the journey. In his class he spoke of journeys: physical, metaphorical, spiritual—it didn't matter. And we read books about journeys on foot, journeys in the mind, even journeys by motorcycle.

He said the point of any journey is the travel, the process of the journey. He said there was no journey whose process is worth forgoing.

My classmates and I politely nodded whenever he said it. But we didn't really believe him.

Yes, yes, the process is important, but the destination, that's the thing, we thought. Whether it was a degree, a career, or merely finishing the long writing assignment for his course, we had our minds on the final destination. If there had been a short cut, a magic way to skip the journey and get to the destination, I think we all would have taken it.

But gradually, my classmates and I began to see the wisdom of his words. The destinations we set our sights on were not always where we wound up. The destinations we set out for didn't always turn out to be places we wanted to be. But the thing of value—no matter the destination—was the process. The process of the journey taught us about ourselves—about who we were, what we stood for, what we needed in life. Most important, the process taught us what we were capable of.

We eventually saw that what we learned from that process could help take us to any destination—any future course we might set for ourselves.

This book is a journey we will take together. But it is a journey we can take only by valuing the process. The destination—a better day, a brighter day—simply does not exist without the process.

The process is reading a daily entry of advice based on the scientific study of living a good life. Each day's entry represents the best information available on living a happy life, a successful life, and a healthy life.

The process is a redefinition of your daily routine.

For most of us, the constants of every day are sleeping and eating. We don't forget either, because they're just too important. Think about it: regardless of pressures at work, regardless of pressures at home, regardless of emergencies that arise, we find time to sleep and eat every single day, because we understand those activities to be at the foundation of our life.

But what would you be capable of if you added time for thought and reflection to your daily foundation? What if every day, regardless of the demands on you, you put aside twenty minutes to think about that day's entry, to think about your life, to think about your journey.

It is this act, this process—simple but revolutionary—that will make progress possible for you. Nothing changes without thought. Nothing improves without thought. No good idea is useful to you—whether one that you read or one that you come up with—unless you have the capacity for thought and reflection.

As children, we had quiet time in school. As adults, we all too often have neither quiet nor time. But no more should thinking be considered a luxury to be sacrificed to a busy day than should sleeping or eating.

Will you end this journey in a better place? Will your destination be a happier place? A healthier place? Yes.

But it is the process of this journey that will make you stronger in every challenge you face—this year, next year, and forever.

SIMPLE SECRETS

FOR BECOMING

HEALTHY,
WEALTHY,
& WISE

Motivation Beats Everything

Lack of motivation is a handicap that can stifle a person's potential regardless of their strengths. If you do not want something, it simply does not matter how talented you are. Understand that motivation is the biggest asset you possess in pursuing your future.

SAM WORKED IN the kitchen washing dishes at a restaurant in Fresno, California. It was undeniably the worst job in the place. "It was back-breaking work in unbelievable heat. The pace was always hectic, and when the dinner rush finally slowed, you had to face the pots and pans," Sam says.

Although only a teenager, Sam thought about the things he would do differently if he ran the restaurant. "The tile floor would get slippery as the night wore on, and we were always trying to come up with ways to keep the waiters from falling down, 'cause if they fell down, it was the dishwashers who had to clean it up," he recalls.

It was only a dream at the time—but little by little he saved what he could. He moved up step-by-step through restaurant jobs until he was running the kitchen. Twenty years after he started as a dishwasher, he opened his first restaurant, and within a few years he had four locations.

Sam, who won an award for the success of his restaurants, credits his outlook for his success: "It would not be possible without hard work, but it would not be possible without believing in it. If I didn't believe, I never would have saved. I never would have learned everything I could about the business. If you have persistence and confidence, you have a bright future."

Researchers found that the future career earnings of schoolchildren were four times more strongly influenced by personal motivation than by any other factor. (Russell and Atwater 2005)

Be Happy to Succeed

We all think we would be happy if we were a success. But happiness is far less dependent on objective measures of success than success is dependent on happiness. A positive approach precedes a positive outcome.

"A LAW FIRM can be a pretty high-stress place," Mike admits. The co-founder of a midsize Indianapolis firm, Mike, together with his partners, committed to a different vision of a law firm from day one.

"We thought you could build a law firm based on the belief that everyone should still have a life," Mike says. No one is expected to make a habit of working late nights or on weekends. Everyone is expected to take the occasional afternoon off to see their child's class play or Little League game. The rules apply equally to the most senior partner and the most junior office assistant.

"You start talking about these things, and some people think this is a firm for slackers," Mike says. "But we're talking about facilitating excellence, not impeding it. We've found that a human approach makes our staff happier, which makes their efforts more sustainable. The great secret here is that we actually expect more of our people, and we get it. Because even though you can get people to work hard under threat and toil, you'll never get them to work their best that way."

Researchers have found that happy individuals are 73 percent more likely to go on to experience positive outcomes in both their career and their personal life. (Lyubomirsky, King, and Diener 2005)

Give Yourself Time

There isn't enough time in the day. We rush around from one thing to the next, not stopping until the day is over. One of the easiest things to cut out of the day to save time is a moment for ourselves. But time spent quietly alone is not a luxury. It is an important component of how we function. Give yourself time to sit, to think, to feel, every single day.

TOLD TO SHUT his eyes and shake his body vigorously, with his limbs gyrating like rubber bands, Kevin began to reconsider whether he should have signed up. "Is this guy for real?" wondered the New York City firefighter as he began Dr. Jim Gordon's program of meditation, yoga, and alternative healing therapies designed to help firefighters deal with the emotional stress of the aftermath of the September 11 attacks.

The workshop was taking place not long after the end of the nine-month cleanup of human remains and debris from the World Trade Center. Kevin meditates and "shakes" stress away nearly every day. "It really calms you down," says Kevin, who is helping Dr. Gordon launch an ongoing program for city firefighters.

But how do you get a firefighter to stretch out on a mat in a yoga pose, meditate to soft music, or learn to breathe steadily—practices initially deemed "ridiculous and crazy" by most first-timers, according to Dr. Gordon. "What we do is, we say, 'Look, you're practical people. Try it for yourselves and see if it makes a difference,'" Dr. Gordon says.

Kevin wants to recruit more of his colleagues to Dr. Gordon's program by explaining to them that it is an independent type of therapy that should appeal to tough-minded firefighters such as themselves. "It's just basic things that you can do to help yourself," Kevin adds.

Researchers found that people who meditated regularly had higher levels of disease-fighting antibodies. (University of Wisconsin 2003)

Creativity Comes from Within

Everyone wants to think of something new—to solve a problem no one else can solve. And every business wants to encourage its employees to have the next great idea. But creativity is not the same as hard work and effort; it requires genuine inspiration. It is the product of a mind thoroughly intrigued by a situation. Thus, creativity comes not when we are paid or rewarded, but when we focus our attention on something because we want to.

JAPAN RAILWAYS EAST had the contract to build a bullet train between Tokyo and Nagano to be put in place in time for the 1998 Winter Olympics.

Unfortunately, the tunnels the company built through the mountains kept filling with water. The company brought in a highly paid team of engineers to come up with the best solution. The engineers analyzed the problems and drew up an extensive set of plans to build an expensive drainage system and a system of aqueducts to divert the water out of the tunnels.

A thirsty maintenance worker one day came up with a different solution when he bent over and took a large swallow of the tunnel water. It tasted great, better than the bottled water he had in his lunch pail.

He told his boss they should bottle the tunnel water it and sell it as premium mineral water.

Thus was born Oshimizu bottled water, which the railroad sells not only from vending machines on its platforms but now also by home delivery.

A huge cost was transformed into a huge profit, all by someone looking at the situation differently.

Studies in which people were offered money in exchange for creative solutions to problems found that monetary rewards were unrelated to peoples' capacity to offer original ideas. (Cooper et al. 1999)

The Mundane Is Heroic

If you are married long enough, the local newspaper will take your picture and write up your story. But that achievement is built on a nearly infinite series of actions, including a daily, hourly, moment-to-moment commitment to each other. It is certainly not always easy, and the rewards are not always immediately apparent, but sacrificing your immediate preferences and committing to sharing, caring, and listening are mundane but heroic steps toward your lifetime relationship goal.

EVEN BEFORE THEY dated, Kathy and William began working out together. Later, after they married, their interest and success in running led them to set a goal of running together in the Boston Marathon. After they had trained for three years together, Kathy's best time qualified her for the race. However, William's did not.

William could have reacted in a variety of ways. He could have wallowed in self-pity. He could have asked Kathy to wait until they could run together. He could have resented his wife's ability to achieve and tried to sabotage her efforts.

"A big part of me wished I was out there running the marathon, of course," admits William. "So what did I do on race day? I went out to five or six locations and cheered her on." William chose to encourage rather than discourage: "I lived vicariously through her. Her success is my success."

William says that in working out together, as in life together, jealousy can invade a relationship, but the most important thing to remember is that "we're a team every day—race day too. We have to be able to give each other the freedom to be able to develop our own talents."

Basic communication skills in a relationship are associated with strong levels of such highly regarded personal qualities as self-restraint, courage, generosity, commitment to justice, and good judgment. (Fowers 2001)

Never Give Up

There are stories we hear about people becoming an overnight success. Of course, it often took decades of anonymous hard work for them to get there. Regardless, success never stops satisfying. Far from losing its power, success late in life is every bit as satisfying as success at a younger age.

FRANK McCOURT TAUGHT writing and literature to New York City high school students.

He dabbled in writing himself. But he'd never published anything.

Central to who he was as person was his experience growing up within his family and his small Irish hometown. It was a life of great sadness, surrounded by poverty and alcoholism, but it was not without its humor and absurdity. Retired from the classroom, Frank committed himself to putting that story on paper.

The result was *Angela's Ashes*, a book that won millions of readers and a Pulitzer Prize.

Frank leaped from total obscurity to international fame. "It's all a big surprise to me, all a big adventure. And I don't know where I'm going. It's a series of shocks," he said shortly after he won the award.

"But it hasn't changed me in any fundamental way," he continued. "I don't have time to get a bloated ego. God knows, I've taken time off, gone into a corner and said, 'OK, ego: bloat!' And it won't."

The capacity to continue trying through repeated setbacks is associated with a 31 percent more optimistic outlook on life and a 42 percent greater life satisfaction. (Meulemann 2001)

See Possibilities Where Others See Obstacles

Even in the strongest relationships, there are reasons for worry. And even in the most tenuous relationships, there are reasons for hope. Constant attention to the weaknesses of any relationship will make every day harder. Constant attention to the strengths of any relationship will make every day a day of possibilities.

THEIRS IS PERHAPS the ultimate example of love and devotion trumping religious differences and the associated political differences. Pam is Jewish, Adil is Muslim, and they have been happily married for more than a decade.

When they met, Adil was interested in asking Pam out on a date but worried she might not want to be involved with a Muslim. "I remember this tension, thinking if I should tell her right away that I am a Muslim," he recalls.

"People are so intense," says Pam. "Everywhere you go, it is 'Jew,' 'Arab,' 'Arab,' 'Jew.' You can't just be." There have been many double takes, criticisms, and insults. Too many to count.

Determined and in love, the couple have worked to straddle the distance between Jewish and Muslim cultures, to exist in the open. In the meantime, symbols and sounds of coexistence permeate their home. Their dining-room armoire displays a Koran next to a menorah. The couple celebrates Jewish holidays alongside Muslim ones.

"If there is anything that our relationship might teach our two worlds, it is compromise," Adil says. "It's the magic word."

An experiment performed with couples who were experiencing conflict had half of the couples discuss the best part of their relationship and the other half discuss the worst aspect of their relationship. Couples discussing the positive side of their relationship reduced their stress levels by 15 percent, whereas those discussing the negative side saw their stress levels increase by 48 percent. (Sullivan 2001)

The Quest for a Perfect Body Is Doomed

Seeking a healthier lifestyle is an inherently good thing that will help you in many ways in your life. But seeking a perfect outcome—the perfect body—is neither good nor helpful. In reality, perfection does not exist, because for every improvement we make, we can always think of something else that could be changed. Seek a healthy body that functions, not a perfect body fit for a display case.

COMEDIAN AND FORMER talk-show host Rosie O'Donnell has battled a weight problem for as long as she can remember. One day Rosie decided to start a club to encourage the overweight to improve their habits and fitness. Seeking a fitness coach, she said, "I didn't want some Barbie-doll type saying, 'You can do it, you can do it.' Anyone who sees that is going to think, 'I'm never going to look like that. Why bother?'"

For the club's head fitness coach, Rosie hired Judy Molnar, who stands six-foot-one and weighs two hundred pounds. "When I first met Judy," Rosie said, "I thought, 'Here's someone who looks like me, looks like a regular person.'" Judy's message—"If I can get fit, anyone can"—resonated with Rosie.

A few years before, Judy began walking for her health. At the time, she weighed three hundred pounds. Gradually her walking routine became a running routine. And although she was not focused on losing weight, it began to happen anyway, "one doughnut at a time," she says. After a year, she had lost one hundred pounds.

When O'Donnell's club sponsored a run, Rosie had a chance to meet countless club members. "These people told me I inspired them," she says. "Well, they inspired me."

Less than 2 percent of people surveyed were unable to come up with something they would want to change about their bodies. (U.S. Department of Health and Human Services 2002)

Don't Let Your First Idea Be Your Only Idea

We begin our careers as almost empty notebooks, and as we progress, our mind fills with notations and observations. Take heed of experience, but realize there are situations where your first lessons no longer apply.

SCHWINN BICYCLE WAS the leader in the industry for one hundred years.

Edward Schwinn, the fourth generation of Schwinns in the business, took control of the bicycle company in 1979. Thirteen years later, the company was on life support, its market share down by 60 percent.

Analysts point to a refusal to live in the present as a reason for the decline of the company. Edward refused outside financing when the company began to show signs of weakness. Because Schwinn was *the* name in bicycles, Edward had refused to spend money on keeping the brand in consumers' consciousness. Because it was always the kind of company that operated on a handshake, Edward agreed to outsource all Schwinn's manufacturing to the same Chinese supplier without adequately protecting the company's long-term interests.

By 1992, Schwinn Bicycle was going under. Product recognition among children had dropped to close to zero. And the Chinese ended their deal with Schwinn and began producing their own bicycles in plants paid for with Schwinn money.

The company declared bankruptcy the same year, and the Schwinn family lost all control over the family's business. Edward Schwinn's explanation for the fall: "We are where we are." To which one family member responded, "Where we are is out of business, because you were asleep at the wheel."

Research on financial managers finds that nine in ten display a particular commitment to sectors in which they experienced their first success. (Goltz 1999)

What You Do Matters

Health is not just a lottery. We are not all just randomly stricken with diseases. Though some health outcomes are completely beyond our control, our likelihood of contracting most diseases is affected by our decisions and behaviors.

KAREN HAS SEEN more than her share of sickness in her family. Both her parents died of cancer, and she agonized as they suffered through its last stages.

She read everything she could on the subject to try to help her parents. "I tried to help, but there were no miracles available," Karen recalls. "But what I did learn is that anyone can drastically reduce their chances of suffering from major diseases like cancer. And I felt I owed it to my parents to try to live a healthy life in their memory."

Karen embraced eating right and exercising as major facets of her life. "It not only makes you healthier, it just makes you feel better," she says. "That's the bottom line."

Karen took up running, hiking, and resistance training. Karen's interest in the subject even led to a midlife career change. She became an exercise physiologist—a person who teaches approaches to exercising.

Karen's work now includes not only teaching exercising to help prevent disease, but also introducing exercise programs to those suffering from cancer, because research shows that exercise improves a patient's prospects for recovery.

Today, she can't imagine living her life any other way. "If I sit at home, then I'm going to feel awful," she says.

Cancer is the number one public health fear. Most people believe that it is impossible or next to impossible to prevent cancer. Researchers have found, however, that half of all cancers can be traced to personal choices such as a sedentary lifestyle, a high-fat diet, prolonged and unprotected exposure to the sun, and tobacco use. (Mayo Clinic 2002b)

There Are Second Chances

Family life is what we make of it—regardless of the form it comes to us in. Whether you are in a traditional family, a stepfamily, or some other type of family situation, you have the capacity to contribute to it and feel loved in it. There are no rules for what makes a family except the ones you make, and there is no time limit on when or how you find a loving family life.

SHARON BROUGHT A son into her second marriage, and her husband brought a daughter. She was anxious about her new blended family, and felt she'd seen and heard mostly misconceptions. "It's seems like it's either *The Brady Bunch* where everything is perfect, or one of those talk shows where a stepfamily comes on and everybody hates each other and everything is a disaster," she says.

Sharon and her family faced many adjustments as they came together. "We decided we were going to look at it as an adventure," she says. "We called ourselves 'the home team.' We didn't want to force the word *family* on the children too soon." But, Sharon adds, within two years of living together, they were thriving. "When the stepfamily comes together, it is like a beautiful extended family from decades ago," she says.

Concerned that many people feel at a loss as to how to approach life as a stepparent, Sharon created *Your Stepfamily,* a magazine of advice, research, and hands-on information. "It's real you-and-me kind of stuff—approachable, touchable stuff," Sharon says.

And the magazine's motto is the same as Sharon's family motto: Embrace the Journey.

Research on stepfamilies finds that participants must accept an often difficult transition period but that ultimately family life satisfaction can be as high in stepfamilies as it is in the most successful traditional families. (Visher, Visher, and Pasley 2003)

Wonder

W̲e all know that daydreaming is for kids. Or it's for the kind of people who don't get anything done. But in truth, giving yourself free time to contemplate whatever might be in your mind puts you on the path to new ideas.

FOR DECADES, THE teachers in West Hartford, Connecticut, have ended class early on Wednesdays. The teachers have homework of sorts—to think about how they can do their jobs better.

Jack, a school-board member, thinks that far too few schools give their teachers the chance to grow on the job. "Most places hire teachers, place them in a classroom, and then that's it," he says. "Nothing to reinvigorate them, nothing to help them refine what they are doing."

Teachers in West Hartford have had the opportunity to learn new classroom techniques, to reshape the curriculum, and to just "expand their horizons," Jack says.

"We have to better understand what productive use of time really is," Jack maintains. "People see teachers out of class, and they think it's a waste of time. But giving a professional a chance to reexamine what they do, giving them a chance to ask questions and exchange information—just giving them time to think about things—is one of the most productive ways to improve their classroom time.

"In my experience, if you just keep doing your job without some time for examination, you don't necessarily get better at the work. You just get more set in your ways."

Scientists have found that the recurring tendency to engage in moments of wonder—to spend time thinking without the structured boundaries of a specific task—leads to 17 percent greater life satisfaction and contributes significantly to creativity. (Lomas 2004)

Volunteer for Yourself

Volunteering for a cause you care about is not only a great benefit to others, but also a great benefit to yourself. Volunteering demonstrates our humanity to ourselves and offers a wonderful opportunity for cultivating feelings of connection to our community. Give of yourself to others, because it is the greatest gift you can give yourself.

THERE ARE TWO reasons Frank spends two days a week volunteering in the Consumer Protection Division of the Maryland attorney general's office. "Number one, it helps people. Number two, it helps me."

Frank deals with citizens who have had consumer disputes with area companies. Frank takes their information and tries to work out an agreement between the customer and the company. "Some of these folks have spent literally everything they have on something they really need—maybe a car, maybe a refrigerator. Then it doesn't work, and the seller says 'Tough.' Or they've signed on for a service they didn't really understand and can't really afford. Now they want to cancel but are told they can't. We step in, try to figure out the basic facts, and try to move the situation forward."

It's not only helping people but working with his mind that Frank values in the experiences. "It keeps me sharp," he says. "Getting all the details. Figuring out the steps. It's a new challenge every time."

Despite the complexities of the task, Frank is no lawyer, and he thinks people imagine they have to be experts to volunteer in his office. "We're looking for people with common sense and life experience here," Frank adds. "If you have that, you could be a valuable volunteer almost anywhere."

Researchers have found that volunteering improves life satisfaction across the generations. Notably, the effect is even greater among those over age sixty, who enjoy 72 percent greater life satisfaction and 54 percent more positive feelings about themselves when they volunteer. (Van Willigen 2000)

Use a Plan, Not a Piecemeal Approach

Your chances of sticking to a health-improvement plan—such as eating right, exercising regularly, or quitting smoking—are higher if you focus on your overall health rather than just the task at hand. Think about the things you could do to improve your health and how they fit together, and each act will reinforce everything else you are trying to do.

SIX YEARS AGO, Lee was hobbling around with a cane. Now the seventy-two-year-old Chicago-area man pumps iron more than two hours a day several times a week. "There was a time when I wasn't in very good shape. I was about fifty pounds too heavy and was loaded with arthritis," he says. But he got tired of living like what he calls an "old man."

Then Lee started to read up on nutrition, exercise, and the aging process. He changed his diet and started exercising. "I have seen so many improvements. I sleep better, have more energy, and my aches and pains went away," he says. "I feel like I'm forty."

Now Lee shares his new enthusiasm for healthy living by speaking to groups in his community. One of his biggest fans is Kristina, who is forty years younger than Lee. "If anyone would have told me a seventy-two-year-old retiree would change my life, I wouldn't have believed it," she says, "but now I know better."

A study compared workplaces where employers provided health, safety, and quitting-smoking programs as one comprehensive service to workplaces where such programs were offered separately. At the end of two years, the investigators found that more than two times as many workers quit smoking and maintained a healthy diet in the comprehensive service than did their counterparts in the separate programs. (Dana-Farber Center for Community-Based Research 2002)

You Have Nothing to Envy in Your Partner

There is no trophy for bettering your partner in the end. The real prize is for accepting that there is no competition with your partner. That prize is contentment and a more satisfying relationship.

WHEN GEORGE BURNS and Gracie Allen first teamed up onstage to perform a comedy act in the 1930s, he had the experience and she was new to the business. The first night, George took the lead and had Gracie feed him the straight lines while he told all the jokes. The act was a disaster.

The next night, George took the straight lines and gave Gracie all the laugh lines. The rest is show-business history. Or, as George Burns put it, "I asked Gracie about her brother, and she talked for the next thirty-eight years."

First onstage, then on radio, and then on TV, the real-life and stage couple played their roles to the hilt, she a befuddled wife, he an exasperated husband. All the while, Gracie was the center of attention, telling the jokes, while George worked the setups for her lines.

For George Burns, standing out of the spotlight in the act while his wife was the center of the show was simply a recognition of ability: "Gracie had a talent the audience loved. I had a talent the audience didn't.

"Gracie got all the laughs," he added, "and that was all right with me, because we split the salaries, and that was good, too."

Married to Gracie for four decades until she passed away, George Burns always wanted her recognized as the star of the show. "Gracie should always have top billing," he said.

People who feel a sense of competition with their partner are 37 percent less likely to feel that their relationship is satisfying. (Romero-Medina 2001)

Resist the Urge to Be Average

Everywhere around you there are average people. They entice you into being more like them by offering their acceptance and by leading you to believe that everyone else is already more like them than you are. But the "average-person sales pitch" leaves out that you will be sacrificing your goals, sacrificing your individuality and unique ideas—leading a life that is not so much yours as it is determined by the preferences of your group.

"A PERSON WHO wants to be a leader must turn his back to the crowd," says the sign on Ty Underwood's desk. Ty runs a job-placement service that works with laid-off workers and the chronically underemployed.

"When I got here, there was an attitude that this was all a show to keep the agency's funding. We'd show up, have the clients come in to fill out some papers, then send them on their way—nobody behaving as if there was important work to be done, nobody behaving as if there was potential to be tapped here."

His first task was to change everything. To two-thirds of the staff, he minced no words: "Here's your resignation. Sign it."

Ty notes that each day begins with one premise: "Everyone who walks through this door can do more. That goes for the counselors and the clients."

In two years, Ty took an office he considered an embarrassment and turned it into a model of effectiveness, with a job-placement record of 71 percent.

Psychologists have observed that bad habits can spread through an office just like a contagious disease. Employees tend to mirror the bad behaviors of their co-workers, with factors as diverse as low morale, poor work habits, and theft from the employer all rising based on the negative behavior of peers. (Greene 1999)

Too Much of a Good Thing Is Too Much

If vitamins are good for us, then more vitamins must be even better for us, right? Nope. It doesn't quite work that way. In some cases, the recommended dosage of a vitamin is all our body can process. In others, taking more than the recommend dosage is harmful. Resist the urge to devise your own supervitamin strategy.

"TAKING TOO MUCH of an essential vitamin or mineral may be as dangerous as going without the nutrient at all," says Dr. Beverly McCabe-Sellers, a professor of dietetics and nutrition at the University of Arkansas for Medical Sciences. She notes the importance of the latest warning from the Institute of Medicine, which for decades has created guidelines on how much of each essential nutrient a person needs. "In the most recent of a series of reports updating nutrients' value to the human body, the institute sets upper limits—the maximum amount an individual may take without risks of adverse health effects—for such things as vitamin A, copper, iron, manganese, and zinc," Dr. McCabe-Sellers notes.

Dr. McCabe-Sellers thinks the report needs to be understood by consumers, because she has seen far too many cases of people "megadosing" on vitamin supplements by taking five or even ten times the recommended dietary allotment for a nutrient.

"Although men require nine hundred micrograms of vitamin A each day and women seven hundred micrograms, some supplements offer as much as seventy-five hundred micrograms in a single dose. That's more than twice the level set by the National Academy of Sciences report as a dangerous overdose.

"This is definitely a situation where you can get too much of a good thing," Dr. McCabe-Sellers says.

People exceeding the recommended daily allowance of vitamins and minerals can worsen the effects of cancer and reduce the effectiveness of conventional cancer therapies. (Dana-Farber Cancer Institute 2002)

It's Never Just One Thing

When we think of attaining success, we often think of achieving a specific goal. But when we land the account, get the promotion, or get a raise, the same nagging concerns that led us to think we desperately needed one more achievement will undermine the value of that achievement. Feelings of success come with the whole of our efforts, our beliefs, our experiences, our lives. Success is based on the total package, not the ribbon on the package.

THEY DON'T TRAVEL in private jets and limousines. There are no roadies to unpack their equipment. They make no outrageous demands for huge dressing rooms or pampered treatment.

The members of Rustic Overtones are just happy to play their alternative rock music in clubs across the country. And when they are finished playing for the night, they pack everything up themselves in their rusty van.

They don't have a contract with a major record company, and much of what they earn for their gigs is used to offset travel expenses.

Will they make it? Drummer Tony McNaboe and the rest of the band certainly hope so, but he explains, "If you don't enjoy every minute of this, then you're in the wrong business. We play for crowds, we play for each other, we'll find a street corner and play for people walking by. We love making music, and whether we get a big record contract and headline a big sold-out show or not, we'll be making music."

Researchers find that people's enduring self-concept—their view of who they are and what they are capable of—is not tied to any single positive or negative event. Instead, a self-concept comprises a combination of beliefs and feelings based on long-term experiences both at home and at work. (Black 1999)

Change Is Possible, Not Easy

Commercials on TV tell you all the time that you can change yourself. In thirty seconds, the commercial actors can get smarter, thinner, prettier, richer. But this fantasy world only sets us up for a fall. When you entered the first grade, you didn't expect to learn a second language, algebra, and the history of the War of 1812 all in the first week. You began an education that took more than a decade and provided you with incredible positive change. Positive change in your life will not be finished today, but it can start today.

CHARLIE'S JOB IS about change. He is brought in to smooth the transition when one company acquires another. It has given him a special perspective on the subject of change.

"Companies have cultures—ways of doing things. These cultures aren't easy to change. Sometimes these cultures hold companies back from doing what they are capable of, and sometimes they make it impossible for two separate businesses to merge and exist together," Charlie says.

What Charlie does is study the cultures of the companies with an eye toward protecting the future: "When you have a culture that is not serving the long-term needs of the company, it needs to be changed. But changed carefully. If you change things too drastically, or change the culture in a negative, threatening way, then there will be high turnover, and you won't have changed the culture as much as destroyed it.

"Healthy change is a long-term process, whether for a company or the people in it."

The decision to make a change offers wonderful feelings of control and optimism, but those are short-lived if the change is not accomplished. Repeated efforts at self-change that are characterized by an expectation of an unrealistically high payoff in an unrealistically short time actually reduce satisfaction with our lives by 40 percent. (Polivy and Herman 2000)

Know Your Health

The less we know about something, the more we are subject to its whim. Not only will knowing more about your health, both when something ails you and when you feel fine, help you live a healthy lifestyle; it will reduce your fears of a health impediment to your quality of life.

FOR BARBARA PARIENTE, being nominated as a justice of the Florida Supreme Court represented an unbelievable triumph, the culmination of a law career during which she encountered few women colleagues. The court hears some of the most controversial cases in the nation, and she holds one of its seven seats.

As a lawyer and as a judge, she never shied away from the challenge of taking on complex cases and understanding countless details. When she found out she had breast cancer, she reacted in the same way. "I wanted to learn everything I could," she says. "The first thing I learned was that you may be fearful, but you will be able to come through it and not only survive, but thrive."

After her initial diagnosis, Barbara threw herself into a mini–medical school curriculum. Barbara received differing advice on how to treat her condition. She took it upon herself to put the advice together and arrive at the best treatment.

For Barbara, getting all the information she could was empowering: "You can say either 'I'm going to give in to this disease' or 'I'm going to confront it and beat it.'" And now, with her cancer in remission, she says, "I can't say I'm glad that I had cancer. But I'm not sad I had cancer. I am healthy. I am surviving. I am thriving."

People who take an active interest not only in their illnesses but in their overall health are 15 percent more likely to feel that their health problems are not reducing their life satisfaction. (Othaganont, Sinthuvorakan, and Jensupakarn 2002)

It's Not How Hard You Try

Trying really hard, by itself, is not a recipe for success in a relationship. In fact, maximum effort can be a great source of frustration and pain when our efforts are not rewarded with a better relationship. Work on your relationship with meaningful goals that will contribute to your relationship's health and your happiness. Work on your relationship with logic and reason, not with maximum effort.

NICOLE HAD PICTURED this day almost her entire life. It was all she had thought about for months. Everything she did was focused on it. It was to be a picture-perfect wedding.

The flowers had been imported from New Zealand. The reception was planned for the Grand Salon of the Essex House in Manhattan. Nicole was wearing a stunning Christoff-designed wedding gown, with a four-carat diamond ring glistening on her left hand.

Everything was set on the wedding day. Except for one small detail: Nicole's fiancé had already left for Tahiti—their honeymoon destination. Without her. The bride's mother watched "as a beautiful wedding turned into a nightmare," said a friend of Nicole's. Nicole soldiered on and attended the reception party for the nonwedding. Then she went about putting her world back in order.

Friends quietly wondered if the wedding fiasco wasn't a case of trying too hard. "Sometimes a man and a woman see marriage differently. They see their relationship to one another differently. A woman may think she's being open in professing her love and pushing the relationship, but the man may just feel pushed," said Nicole's friend. "Nicole needed to pace the relationship. You can go too fast and try too hard."

People who said they were trying hard to improve their relationship were 33 percent less likely to be happy than were people who said they were putting some effort in improving their relationship. (Hairston 2001)

You Can't Force Yourself to Like Broccoli

Personalities are not unlike shoe sizes: they are not subject to our choice or preference, but they can occasionally be fudged—with uncomfortable consequences. Some people can speak before large audiences and be exhilarated by the experience, whereas others would be petrified. Some people can study an equation for years and be fascinated by it, whereas others would instantly long for human interaction and variety. Realize who you are, what your true personality is—and choose a future that fits.

HARDLY A DAY goes by without at least one of his clients refusing to work with him. In fact, sometimes they spit up on him.

But photographer Jean Deer loves his job.

He has taken hundreds of children's portraits, and he is well acquainted with all the tricks of the trade to make a baby smile. Jean is an expert in every funny face and noise imaginable.

"When it's over, everyone—me, the parents, and the children—are exhausted, but that's usually a good sign," Jean says.

Jean found that getting babies to flash their smiles wasn't the only way to get a great picture, and that a grumpy baby was just another source of inspiration. "I was taking a photo once of this infant who literally wanted nothing to do with me. He would not look up, just stared at the floor," Jean recalls. Jean got down on the floor with him, took the picture from a perspective he'd never used before, and wound up with one of the best photographs he'd ever taken.

The job requires two major traits, Jean believes: "Not everyone can just hang out a shingle and call himself a photographer. It's all a matter of being patient and being energetic and then capturing the right moment."

Even as people experience different phases of their lives, their underlying personality remains constant after about age sixteen. (Barto 1998)

The Past Is Not the Future

Your relationship past is not your relationship future. Your relationship future is not limited by your experiences of the past or by your disappointments of the past. You can learn from your experiences and avoid the mistakes of the past.

MONICA SELES KNOWS she will always be measured against her younger self, the one who turned tennis professional at fifteen and claimed the number one ranking a little more than two years later.

Her storybook career turned tragic when a deranged man burst from the stands and stabbed her while she was playing in the 1993 German Open. "I got stopped at the height of my career," Monica says.

The painful journey back to the tennis court changed her perspective: "Every day you play, you win some, you lose some. If you treat people based on how you did on the tennis court, which a lot of players do, you'll wind up throwing away your personal life. My theory is to get up and try again in every way, in every aspect of my life—in my tennis career, in my personal life. I try to just keep going on."

Monica embraces the notion that she can make a positive change in her life. "I don't believe you can ever be what you were because of so many things, your experiences," she says. "You cannot be the same person. I live in the present."

Most people who left an unhappy relationship were in a happy relationship within three years, and 74 percent said that their new relationship was significantly different. (Sweeney 2002)

Competence Starts with Feeling Competent

D on't wait for your next evaluation to improve your judgment of yourself, because feelings are not dependent on facts. Feelings of competence actually start with the feelings; the competence itself follows.

ROSS, A DANCER from Springfield, Missouri, has dreams of making it to Broadway.

His road to dancing glory began with local amateur productions—productions in which auditions take place in front of all the other performers trying out. Ross found the experience daunting; it was like being examined by a doctor with all your peers watching. "I was so scared. I felt like I had just come out of the cornfields," Ross says.

Sometimes he succeeded, and sometimes he didn't. But Ross was able to try out for different parts in various productions, and he gained tremendously from the experience: "I have more confidence about my auditioning technique now that I have done it in front of so many people, so many times."

When he tried out for a professional touring company for the first time, he won a spot in a production of *Footloose*.

Ross has one explanation for his immediate success in landing a professional part: "I had confidence. If you want to do it, you have to really want it and believe in it. You have to make it happen. You can't sit back and hope that someone is going to help you along."

For most people in one study, the first step toward improving how they did their job had nothing to do with the job itself; rather the first step was improving how they felt about themselves. In fact, for eight in ten people in the study, self-image mattered more in how they rated their job performance than did their actual job performance. (Gribble 2000)

We're Too Good at Imagining the Worst-Case Scenario

When something is wrong with us, we can easily imagine the worst outcome. The doctor will tell us how horrible our situation is and how horrible the recommended treatment is. This process of exaggerating the threat to ourselves not only creates anxiety but also has the dangerous effect of encouraging us not to seek treatment. Don't let yourself get caught in a guessing game that does you no good. Acknowledge what you don't know, and get the answers from a medical professional.

WHY DO SO many people with medical needs avoid going to see a doctor? "That's the biggest question for all of us," says Dr. Ed Hayer of South Carolina.

"'The doctor says' is an awfully weighty phrase," adds Dr. Hayer. "There's a feeling that the news the doctor brings will never be good, that the answers will be painful, and that knowing their fate would be a terrible burden."

In Dr. Hayer's field, cardiac medicine, this feeling can be disastrous: "We can do so much more the earlier we see a patient with heart problems. And fear is one of the major obstacles to our seeing patients when we need to. What can happen is that fear of a terrible diagnosis actually helps create the terrible diagnosis, because if the patient had not been fearful and had come in sooner, their outcome would be better."

Dr. Hayer's advice for those who are worried about seeking medical care is to understand that you will always be in control. "No one will force a treatment on you. You are free to walk away, to seek a second opinion," Dr. Hayer says. "But we're here to help you."

In a study of those who suffer back pain, researchers found that people were ten times more likely to think surgery was necessary than was actually the case. (University of Michigan 2002a)

Set Rules for Conflict in Your Relationship

You are never going to agree with your spouse or partner on everything, and you shouldn't try to. But you must level the playing field in your discussions by deciding how you can air concerns to each other in a format that allows both of you to be open.

JAMES LEIJA KNOWS a thing or two about conflict. He's a professional boxer, among the best in the lightweight class. "Although I box, I hit people, I do it within the rules," he says. "You have to have rules—or you have no sport." James lives his life by the same standard.

James and his wife, Lisa, were high school sweethearts before getting married. They have no wedding-day photos because James was still black and blue from U.S. Olympic boxing trials on the big day.

Their first years were lean. James turned pro but barely made enough money to pay for his training expenses. Lisa worked as a receptionist and paid for everything else.

The break finally came when James won a fight against a top contender. By the time he had claimed the world junior lightweight title, he was rich beyond his imagination.

Now, instead of money worries, they had to deal with groupies. Women just threw themselves at him during autograph sessions. Before the couple could argue over it, James thought about Lisa's feelings and decided to avoid places where he would draw too much attention.

"This is a sport where divorce is as common as blood in the ring," James's manager points out. "But James and Lisa have figured out how to put each other first."

When both partners in a relationship employ the same strategy for dealing with disagreements, they experience 12 percent less conflict and are 31 percent more likely to report that their relationship is satisfying. (Pape 2001)

Give Yourself the Best Chance to Eat Well

People will eat what's available to them. If you don't regularly buy junk food, how often are you going to want a chip so badly that you're willing to walk to the store and buy a bag? On the other hand, if you make healthy foods easily available, the likelihood of choosing a piece of fruit for a snack rises dramatically. Be strategic about your food choices when you are not hungry, and you will be much more health oriented when you are.

GLORIA KNOWS ABOUT the importance of eating habits. As a physician, she advises patients about nutrition. As a person, she struggles to eat right and maintain a healthy weight.

"I come from a long line of really big women. I was destined to be big," she says. And while she rejects drastic diets, she knows and lives with the importance of eating right for her health.

Gloria's house is full of fruit, available anytime for her four children. Junk-food snacks are absent. And she and her kids eat a home-cooked meal every night to reduce the temptations of large sizes and unhealthy foods that they would find in a restaurant.

"Would I prefer it if I had lived my life at, like, 125 pounds? Well, yeah, definitely," she says. "But we have to start swapping the way we see things. We have to get away from the blame and the shame, all the worry, and get focused on health. And the way to do that is to surround yourself with what you should have, and keep what you shouldn't out of reach."

Researchers found that for every additional supermarket in their neighborhood, people become 32 percent more likely to eat their recommended daily portion of fruits and vegetables. Researchers attribute this result to an increased ease of access to affordable and nutritious foods. (University of North Carolina 2002b)

You Are Never Too Old to Improve Your Habits

I t's too late to improve my health." Many people think just that—that their habits are set and that even if they could change them, what good would it do? In fact, improving your habits can improve your health at any age. There's no value in lamenting what you didn't do for yourself in the past, but there is tremendous value in thinking about what you can do for yourself now and in the future.

RICHARD DOESN'T CALL himself a senior citizen. And those who have seen him compete in triathlons probably wouldn't call him that, either.

At sixty-six, he has won his age division in eight triathlons, sometimes finishing ahead of men half his age. The triathlons include a four-hundred-meter swim, followed immediately by a twenty-kilometer bicycle ride, followed immediately by a five-kilometer run.

One of the trickiest parts of a triathlon, according to Richard, is the transitions, especially when you have to get out of the water and into your bike equipment. Because the clock never stops, "you just have to try to go as fast as you can," he says.

"My last triathlon had about two hundred competitors. It was fun to be one of the fastest ones. This one was open to anyone over fifty. There was a man and a woman, between seventy-five and eighty years old, who did the triathlon. There was also an eighty-six-year-old woman who did it as a relay with her sixty-two-year-old son," Richard says.

Richard has no plans to slow down or give up triathlons: "I believe age is just a number and life is what you make it."

Researchers found that those over age seventy-two who increased their frequency of exercise improved their overall health, had a better outlook on life, and enjoyed a 20 percent longer life span. (Case Western Reserve University 2002)

A Victory at All Costs Is Not a Victory

Attempting to succeed in every single thing you do, to win every disagreement, and to get to do everything your way would lead you to a myopic focus on meaningless confrontations instead of a big-picture focus on what you really want.

KI SUH PARK is one of the leading architects in Los Angeles. He accepts nothing less than total effort from himself. And he demands total effort from those around him. He was known for setting records for firing people and insulting colleagues when he returned their memos to them with grammatical errors highlighted.

When Los Angeles suffered through the violence and destruction of the riots of 1992, his perspective began to change. Ki Suh was asked to lead Rebuild L.A.—an initiative to both replace destroyed buildings and reinvigorate the economy of impoverished sections of Los Angeles.

The experience changed his perspective dramatically. "I used to look through my eyes on everything, form an opinion from my eyes. But I learned that you really have to have empathy for other people, how they see the same thing," he says.

When he took on the project of helping Los Angeles, he was suddenly thrust into thinking about the big picture. His purpose has changed, from getting everything done his way to making a contribution to what needs to be done. When new projects—projects that reflect his vision as well as the wishes of the community—open, though, "it is," says Ki Suh, "exhilaration."

The will to succeed comes in two distinct forms. Hypercompetitive people (about 60 percent of competitive people) focus on winning all the time, regardless of the importance of the matter. Self-oriented competitive people (about 40 percent of competitive people) focus on doing well, but with an emphasis on improving themselves so that they can do even better in the future. (Glaman 1999)

You Have to Have Art

When many of us sort out the essentials of life from the luxuries of life, artistic things fall on the luxury side. But art can change our outlook, our reality. Art represents imagination and possibility. And whether it's something you create or just something you observe, there should be art in your life.

DENISE TAKES A little time each week for painting. From her youngest days, Denise felt most at ease with a paintbrush in her hand. "We didn't have much. In fact, it seemed we had less than just about everybody I knew," she says. "But the times I felt good about myself were the times I spent creating."

School didn't hold her interest at first. Denise dropped out of high school repeatedly before coming back later to pursue a high school degree and then a college degree. Even though she didn't study art in school, art helped give her the confidence to try again.

"We need to have some reason to believe in ourselves," Denise says. "We need to have some outlet for the emotions we feel but can't express. I had those things in painting."

Today her favorite paintings are displayed in her living room, while much of her work remains stored in closets. Talking about and showing her work is something she's only recently begun: "A friend asked me for a painting I had done that she saw leaning against the wall—it's actually kind of a self-portrait, but it's from an angle, so you wouldn't know it. It made me think about sharing more of what I've done. Maybe it will do someone else some good, too."

Regular exposure to art—whether it be our own efforts to create something, an object we bought to hang on the wall, or regular trips to a museum—is associated with a 7 percent increase in life satisfaction. (Michalos 2005)

Accomplish Something Every Day

Sometimes days fly by without anything standing out in your mind, without any tangible improvement. Every day make sure, no matter how small the effort, that you do something to make your dreams come true.

CHARLIE WORKS WITH children with severe attachment disorder. These children's brains leave them in a heightened state of alert at all times, regardless of what is going on around them. Caused by trauma or neglect at very early stages, severe attachment disorder causes children to have trouble functioning in any number of settings, including school, and such children are prone to reject attachments to caregivers or others they might come in contact with.

Charlie, a physical therapist, is taking part in a new wave of treatment that tries to create moments of calm in lives of endless havoc. He works with a neurofeedback machine that measures brain waves. When the child maintains a calm state, the child is rewarded with a simple game to play on the computer screen. Over the course of weeks, the amount of calm time required to activate the game increases, gradually helping children attempt to control their emotions.

Charlie says that the children "learn to like the feeling of calm they get. By challenging the brain, much as you challenge your body in physical exercise, we can help your brain learn to function better.

"It's a struggle. There is no overnight cure or magic pill. But every day they can get a little closer to where they can make it in a classroom, make it through their day. It makes you realize that whatever you're trying to do, there is room to try to get better every single day."

People who thought they were making progress toward their goals—regardless of how much they still had left to accomplish—were 51 percent more likely to be satisfied with themselves than people who felt they were stagnating. (DeShon and Gillespie 2005)

You Must Approve of Yourself

You can make the best plans in the world for your life. But no action, no accomplishment, no outcome will offer you ultimate fulfillment. You must offer yourself complete, unconditional approval regardless of whatever takes place in your life.

TWO OF FREDDY Johnson's good friends have gone on to become famous and well-paid head coaches in professional and college basketball. Freddy coaches high school boys' basketball on a far smaller stage, for a far smaller paycheck.

Far from being jealous of his friends or disappointed in himself, Freddy celebrates their successes and his own. He keeps newspaper clippings about his old friends in his office for his players and visitors to see.

And Freddy never doubts the value of spending almost three decades teaching and coaching the game of basketball. "It's amazing where some of the guys I know are now," he says. "But I'm happy where I am, too. I wouldn't trade it for the world." Freddy has won more than six hundred games and half a dozen state titles.

Freddy's fellow high school coaches admire his willingness to keep learning and his willingness to surround himself with good people. "Head coaches always want to be the dominant force on their team," says one competitor. "No one else should know as much as they do. No one else should question decisions that are made. But Freddy seeks to be around the best assistants in the game because he has the self-confidence to surround himself with talented people and to take their success as something he, too, can be proud of."

Those who considered themselves a success were 25 percent less likely to feel anxious about their lives, 14 percent less likely to be selfish, and 45 percent more likely to say they enjoyed their lives. (Chamberlain and Haaga 2001)

Healthy Living Is an Attitude

What is the difference between someone who has healthy habits and someone who doesn't? It's not ability. Anyone could choose to eat better foods or avoid unhealthy habits. It's not inclination. Everyone would prefer being healthy to the alternative. It is, however, attitude. Specifically, an optimistic view of one's ability to engage in healthy habits is the most important ingredient in actually following those healthy habits.

SUE HIT THE WALL in the spring of 2001.

At age forty, Sue, a mother of three, had tried dieting for years. She was used to zippers not zipping and buttons not buttoning. But the icing on the cake that motivated her to drop seventy pounds? Not finding a dress at the mall.

"I couldn't find anything that fit me in the stores," says Sue, who made up her mind that day to lose weight.

"Losing the weight is just the beginning," she says. "Keeping it off is the hard part. It's a lifestyle change. You can't go back to your old habits."

Sue thinks most people are overwhelmed before they even start. "They think it will be too hard, that they are not strong enough to make a change. But I found that you can do this in small steps," Sue says. "If you have the right attitude about your family, your work, and your health, you can see that everything in your life is interconnected, and that the reason you can succeed in health is the same reason you can succeed in anything you care about doing."

Doctors conducted a study of recently pregnant women and found that the single best predictor of their eating and exercise habits after pregnancy was not their physical condition or their weight, but their belief in their ability to take care of themselves. (Cornell University 2001)

Write Down the Directions

If you were going to take a complicated journey out of town, you would write down the directions. But if you were considering the future path of your life, your goals, and what you needed to do to achieve them, you probably wouldn't write any of it down. Think of it—the most significant journey of your life, and you probably won't put a word of the directions on paper. Putting your plans, goals, and ideas on paper makes them more real for you, more tangible. Every step you take to define what you want and what you need to do to get it increases the chances that you will actually pursue these goals and someday achieve them.

HARRY IS A career counselor who works with professionals from various fields who feel unfulfilled.

Harry doesn't just ask them what it is they really want. He asks them, "What's your quest?" He works with people to explore not just what they want to do, but what they need to do.

Harry often finds people unprepared to answer his question. "You ask people what they really need to do, and it strikes most of them as a question they either haven't thought about or gave up thinking about a long time ago," he says.

Harry asks the people he counsels to keep a journal, because he believes that in their journal their true quest will come to light. "If you write down whatever comes to you, you will be able to see the patterns of your thoughts, discover things you didn't even know about yourself, and discover how you fit into your quest," he adds.

People who regularly keep a journal or some kind of written record pertaining to their aspirations are 32 percent more likely to feel that they are making progress in their lives. (Howatt 1999)

It's the Little Things That Matter the Most

The peaks of life may be wonderful, and the depths painful, but the average day is neither. We define our relationships on the basis not of the best days or the worst days—but the average days. Strive to be supportive in average ways on average days, and you will have put in place a major building block of your relationship's foundation.

BILL AND KELLY and their five children live on the 250-acre farm where Bill grew up working the land with his father.

The stresses of farming have taken a toll. Large bills and a low return for crops had left Bill sullen one minute, raging the next.

"I'd blow up easy over little things," he says. "Something is out of place, I'm angry about it. Something is not done, I'm angry about it." Like many farmers, Bill resisted the idea of seeking help. He was proud and independent—tough enough to handle his own problems, or so he thought.

"But I look out my window and wonder, 'What am I going to do to get more land so that I can make a living?' and there weren't any answers. So I just took it out on the people around me," he says.

Bill received counseling from a Minnesota state program that began as a means of offering agricultural advice and was later expanded to deal with the great personal stress many farmers were experiencing.

Bill says he's learning how to deal more effectively with stress: "I don't get angry like I used to. I think before I react to things. I put things in perspective."

Interviews with longtime married couples revealed that nine in ten defined their marriage not in relation to the best and worst events of their lives, but in relation to typical interactions and typical events. (Appleton and Bohm 2001)

Couch Time Affects Body and Mind

Rest is a crucial part of our lives—but it cannot become the central part of our lives. Too much time on the couch or the recliner degrades the ability of our bodies and minds to function. They require regular use to continue functioning.

MARY RAKED IN the winnings as the top scorer among the bridge players at the Beachwood Community Center in northeastern Ohio. "I made a killing," she says, smiling, recalling how she scooped up $6.50 in coins. But that's not why she plays. "It keeps your mind going," she says.

Mary may not know it, but new research may prove she's on to something. Playing bridge, or taking part in any kind of social and intellectual activity, really does keep the mind going—and with it, the body.

Neurologist Dr. Robert Friedland of Case Western Reserve University School of Medicine says that "there is a growing number of studies supporting the theory that an active mind keeps the brain and body healthy. The brain is like any other organ in the body. It ages better, with more health and better function, when it is used."

The thinking brain is like a star athlete: through regular practice it can simply outperform. And any kind of activity that uses the brain can fortify it. Learn a musical instrument, take a Shakespeare class, study Portuguese, Dr. Friedland says. And for Mary and her friends, that means keeping the cards coming.

Researchers tracked almost two thousand people age sixty-five and older over seven years. Those who engaged in leisure activities that required active brain use—such as reading, playing a game, even just talking with friends—reduced their risk of Alzheimer's by 38 percent. Conversely, the more time people spent in inactive pursuits—such as lounging on the couch—the slower their brain response was and the weaker their immune system became. (Columbia University 2003a)

Winners Are Made, Not Born

The great successes of our time are just extraordinary people whom fate smiled on. Aren't they? In truth, people who get ahead get where they are by strategically following a pattern that produces success. They learn what it takes to get ahead. We understand that to build a house it take a plan, a blueprint. But we sometimes forget that to build a successful life it also takes a blueprint.

CHEF WALTER POTENZA owns three thriving Italian restaurants in Rhode Island.

He studied and trained to be a chef, but he sees now that his abilities are the product of a lifetime education. When he opened his first restaurant, "all of a sudden my schooling, the knowledge and the history of my family, the respect and ethics of my father came into play," he says. "It made me an academic, a person who explored the food business."

And the learning never stops. "One of the secrets is, it's a business where you constantly need to stay on top. Chefs are not born," he says. Walter explains that the process continues for him every day: "I'm an obsessive reader. Every time you read a book, you get ideas. Then you introduce your ideas in your workplace. You make more work for yourself."

And success in the cooking business is something he has a clear definition of: "The success that I would like to have is to be remembered as a man who was innovative, who believed in authenticity and the culture of Italian cuisine in America. Food is the link to the past and to family."

Case studies of business executives reveal that 98 percent see their position as the result of plans and strategy and that more than 50 percent credit using a successful person as an example to help define that plan. (Gordon 1998)

See the Love Around You

We are sometimes quick to see the problems in our day and reluctant to focus on the joy in our lives. Regardless of your relationship status, think of the many people who love you and of the depth of their love for you. Feeling loved and knowing that you are worthy of love are necessary to creating or maintaining any relationship.

LANCE AND REBECCA were already married with a son when Lance enrolled in law school. A professor warned that law school life had ended more marriages than he could count. When he graduated, Lance was the only student in his class still married to the same person.

It wasn't easy. "There were days when he'd go to school and I'd just cry," Rebecca says. "I felt like Lance was in law school and I was knee-deep in diapers. But that there wasn't really a 'we.'"

Their relationship continued in a state of wedded mediocrity after law school. Then, eight years later, a doctor told Rebecca she had a terminal disease.

"I withdrew, even though that's when Rebecca needed me more than ever," Lance says. "Because I couldn't face life without her."

Eventually, another doctor caught the misdiagnosis, and Rebecca's health improved. The emotional healing, however, took longer.

"I know I'm loved, and I will always be loved. And Lance is trying harder to show it in all kinds of ways," Rebecca says.

Lance thinks he understands better now. "Rebecca has always been there for me," he says. "That is the definition of romance. To love so much that you are always there. She made me feel loved. I have to show her my feelings, too."

People in satisfying relationships were 22 percent more likely to think of themselves as well loved by family members and friends than were people in unsatisfying relationships. (Sprecher and Felmlee 2000)

The Cold Doesn't Give You a Cold

Button up or you'll catch cold." Age-old advice we've all heard. But temperature does not cause colds. Colds are caused by viruses transmitted person to person. The best way to prevent getting a cold is to wash your hands to prevent the spread of the virus through contact.

THE SICKNESS WE call a cold is called a cold in most languages of the world. The idea that being cold can give you a cold has been widely held for centuries. Yet science has found no evidence for this belief.

One of the first studies on the matter more than a half century ago took a group of volunteers and exposed half to warm temperatures and half to cold. There was no difference in their likelihood of their catching a cold. Indeed, we know today that colds are common at every latitude and longitude in the world, from the deserts to the Arctic.

Some of the most interesting studies on the subject have come from small, isolated communities such as island villages. Among these studies is a 1931 field study of Longyear City, an Arctic coal-mining settlement midway between the Norwegian mainland and the North Pole. For seven months of the year, the town's five hundred residents were iced in, and during that time colds were almost nonexistent. However, the arrival in port of the first ship of summer invariably brought with it a full-blown cold epidemic, leading researchers to conclude that being cold, by itself, is irrelevant to catching a cold.

Researchers found that more than 50 percent of people surveyed thought they could catch a cold by not wearing a coat in winter. Almost 60 percent believed chilly weather could cause a cold. Less than 10 percent correctly identified viruses as the transmitters of colds. (University of Texas Southwestern Medical Center 2002a)

Anticipate Irrationality

We understand the nature of a problem, and we carefully contemplate an ideal solution. Everyone should see how great an idea it is, and there should be no opposition. Unfortunately, we often make an assumption of rationality in others. A good idea will be supported because it is a good idea. Experience eventually teaches us that those around us will make irrational decisions. Be prepared not only to sell your ideas in response to legitimate questions, but also to overcome the ill-conceived fears that others may express.

WORLD-RENOWNED ECONOMIST John Maynard Keynes used to explain what the stock market is really about by comparing it to a contest that British newspapers used to run.

Contestants were given dozens of photographic portraits and asked to choose the six faces that other people would think were the most beautiful. The person whose answers most closely matched the collective opinion of the other contestants was the winner.

"It is not a case of choosing those which, to the best of one's judgment, are really the prettiest, nor even those which average opinion genuinely thinks the prettiest. We have reached the third degree, where we devote our intelligences to anticipating what average opinion expects the average opinion to be," Keynes once wrote in an economics article. In this game or in the stock market, Keynes argued, the task wasn't to figure out what was rationally best. Instead, the game and the stock market reflect the beliefs, ridiculously flawed though they may be, of the average person anticipating what other average people might do.

Research on the hiring process shows that a fear-based concern, often of the consequences of hiring a person who is too talented, is a factor in more than 20 percent of hiring decisions, despite there being no strategic or rational basis for such a concern. (Baker 2000)

Attitude Triumphs over Outcome

People can get discouraged easily. We want something badly—and when we can't seem to get it, we can lose hope. But the world is changing every day. You are changing every day. There is no way to predict exactly what will happen or when it will happen. What you can do is continue.

ELLEN HAS LIVED and worked in New York City for almost a decade. She says looking for a relationship in the city can be harder than finding a seat on the subway at rush hour.

"There's not a lot of warmth, because people are in a hurry," Ellen says. "People are putting in long hours, and it's hard to make a transition to being social."

Ellen has not given up. In fact, she's convinced things can only get better. "Five years ago, I was getting pretty serious with a guy I was dating," she recalls. "After we dated a few months, he told the building manager he was my husband, and they gave him the key to my apartment.

"He took jewelry, camera equipment, found the keys to my car, and drove my stuff away in it."

Fortunately for Ellen, he also stole one more thing: "He took a pair of concert tickets. They were really good seats. That's how the cops found him. In my seats at a rock concert at Madison Square Garden. With another woman.

"I'm glad I have a positive outlook. I get a good laugh out of all this. I don't let it bother me, I just keep on dating."

In long-term studies of people over the course of decades, the capacity to ultimately find a happy relationship was not affected by the timing of love relationships earlier in life but was affected by the person's attitude toward their experiences. (Werner and Smith 2001)

The Best Defense Is to Listen

Nobody likes to be criticized. Unfortunately, defensiveness does not serve you. It encourages you to ignore potentially useful feedback, which inhibits your ability to improve. Know that you are capable, and show it. But do not fight criticism merely because you can.

ED MADE IT to the executive level. He was vice president of sales for a well-established communications company.

A bad year in sales hit the company hard, and layoffs reached all the way to senior management personnel. Ed found himself sending out résumés for the first time in twenty years.

What he experienced was all manner of rejection—from being completely ignored to being told he was overqualified for the positions he applied for. "I could do some of these jobs in my sleep. I couldn't believe I was sitting in front of some pipsqueak in human resources needing their approval," Ed says.

"My friends were sympathetic, but they told me I needed a new attitude," he recalls. "Knowing I should have these jobs, and then treating the process as if it was beneath me, was not going to convince anyone I was the right person for the job.

"They were right, and until I got past what I felt like doing and began to see what I should be doing, I didn't get anywhere."

Ultimately Ed, and his new approach to things, landed a job—ironically enough, in human resources.

Defensiveness is negatively correlated with learning on the job. People with highly defensive personality traits speak more times in meetings, are more likely to interrupt a speaker, and are one-fourth slower in adapting to new tasks. (Haugen and Lund 1999)

Always Being Right Is Wrong for Your Health

People with a very high estimation of themselves and little respect for others wind up experiencing more stress and anger as they deal with a world that constantly disappoints them. Thinking yourself always right is neither a helpful social trait nor a sound health habit. See the value in other people's perspectives, even if you highly value your own.

"FEELING THAT YOU are better than everybody else, or feeling that you are always right, might seem empowering. But really it's mostly isolating. It leads to a tremendous amount of tension," says Dr. James Coyne, a professor of psychiatry at the University of Pennsylvania.

The medical implications are great, he adds: "We've seen everything from tooth decay to ulcers to heart problems linked to this very basic ability to get along."

In addition to avoiding medical problems, the ability to feel connected to others aids the recovery process from disease. "Even when your own determination to get better wavers, the connections to others put you back on track," Dr. Coyne says.

Ultimately, bullheadedness can turn into a matter of life and death, according to Dr. Coyne's work. Dr. Coyne and his colleagues videotaped heart patients' arguments in their homes and grouped them according to the negativity of their interactions. Those heart patients who were more negative toward the other person in arguments were 1.8 times as likely to die within four years as those who were less negative. "That's powerful stuff," Dr. Coyne says.

Researchers found that 62 percent of absolutist thinkers—people with a very high opinion of themselves and a low tolerance for compromise—suffered from high levels of anger and stress, which depressed the functioning of their immune systems. (University of Bradford 1999)

How We See the World
Is More Important Than How the World Is

What is the shape of the world? What condition is it in? Scientists, philosophers, and kings could offer a never-ending debate on these questions. But there is no real grade for the world apart from the one you assign it.

URBAN WORD NYC is a nonprofit organization dedicated to teaching poetry to New York City youngsters. The group places visiting poets in local public schools to expose young people to poetry and to give them a chance to try writing. Students can also visit the center to participate in poetry workshops and work with mentors, many of whom originally became interested in poetry through the Urban Word program. The group's poetry competition draws hundreds of entrants.

Urban Word teaches the rules of rhyme, meter, and flow, but also teaches the biggest rule of all: the only rules for your poetry are those you choose to follow. "We break down barriers to poetry. In school, poets are dead men from three hundred years ago. We show them that every time and every place has poetry. There are poets here among us," says Michael, a director of the program.

Many of the aspiring poets share their words in poetry slams—a combination poetry reading and performance piece in which the words are giving a full dramatic performance. Maya, a young poet in the program, writes about race and life in the city.

"This is a tool for life. Maya takes the challenges she faces on an everyday basis, and breathes an artistic life into speaking of them. And she comes out of it with discipline, composure, and courage," Michael says.

Research comparing people with a strong sense of satisfaction to those with low levels of satisfaction finds that they have objectively similar lives. (Miner, Glomb, and Hulin 2005)

Express Your Love

My loved ones know that I love them. How could they not? I feel love for them all the time. But even if the love you feel is obvious to you, your family still needs to hear it. We often assume that people, especially those who are close to us, know what we are thinking and feeling and that therefore we don't need to keep affirming our love and affection. The truth is that doubts spring up, even if they are not rational, and that all family members are reassured when you share your feelings of love for them.

TONYA GREW UP in a big family, sharing a home with brothers, sisters, and cousins. But she says she never doubted her place in it. "Every day, my mother said she loved me. Every single day," Tonya says. It was a very powerful lesson. "There were a lot of mouths to feed, and times that we struggled. But you never felt unwanted, or overlooked, because there was always a hug coming, always a smile."

Tonya says the joy of family life is something she's made a central part of her parenting. "People always look forward to going places, doing exciting things," she says. "When I go places, I look forward to getting back home. When I see my girls, I'm like a flower in bloom." She says a happy, healthy family "is all I could wish for" and that showing her family her love for them is her "reason for being here."

She admits that being a mother takes a lot of effort and dedication: "Your job is never done. But it's the best job in the world."

———————————

People are 47 percent more likely to feel close to a family member who frequently expresses affection than to a family member who rarely expresses affection. (Walther-Lee 1999)

Eat Your Spinach

Foods rich in folic acid, or folate, help reduce the risk of stroke and heart disease. Eating two servings a day of such foods, including tomatoes and leafy green vegetables such as spinach and romaine lettuce, decreases levels of an amino acid that contributes to the disease process that underlies heart disease and stroke.

DESPITE ITS HIGH nutrient content, and Popeye's best efforts, most people don't ask for spinach every day. But researchers at the University of Arkansas have found a simple solution: put spinach instead of iceberg lettuce on your sandwiches. Even better, they've found that you can't taste the difference.

Marjorie Fitch-Hilgenberg, a professor of nutrition at the university, has been working on a project intended to slip a little more nutrition into food. "We know that people don't eat the recommended number of servings of vegetables, and as a result, they're missing out on the nutrients these vegetables provide," Professor Fitch-Hilgenberg says. "With spinach, we realized we could make a small change to the food people already eat and have a significant impact on their nutritional status."

When Professor Fitch-Hilgenberg and her colleagues tested their idea by secretly replacing iceberg lettuce with spinach in a variety of sandwiches, none of the tasters seemed to suspect the switch. "Only one or two people mentioned that the lettuce looked very green," Professor Fitch-Hilgenberg says.

Professor Fitch-Hilgenberg says she's made the switch at home. "I've had no complaints."

People who consumed at least two servings of folate-rich foods per day had a 20 percent lower risk of stroke and a 13 percent lower risk of cardiovascular disease. Unfortunately, only 32 percent of American adults are getting enough folate per day. (Tulane University 2002)

Don't Be Bound by Tradition

For a relationship to function and thrive, we must live within our own standards, not those imposed upon us from another time.

JAIME THOUGHT HE was a good husband and father. He worked long days, but his work paid for life's necessities. On days off, his attitude was "Don't bother me."

Jaime says that his experience is all too common: "From my father, to myself, to my friends, Latino dads find it hard to express positive emotion—to tell their wife how wonderful she is or to show their kids they are making you proud.

"Finally I said, 'No more. I want my wife and children to come to me, to be happy when I come home.'"

Jaime's new perspective came with his involvement in Los Padres, a Colorado-based group of Latino dads devoted to improving communication with their wives and children. They hold classes and regular meetings to share a message of family commitment.

"In Los Padres, we are redefining 'macho,'" Jaime explains. "Being a real man, a family man, means communicating, not wanting to be left alone. Being a man means getting down on the floor and playing with your child. It means never being afraid to show love."

Jaime's involvement in Los Padres has changed his life, and his family's life. "I appreciate what great gifts have been given to me, and I make sure my family knows that," he says.

Studies of relationships find that both men's and women's expectations have changed significantly in less than a generation. Today, partners in happy, long-term relationships are three times more likely to embrace a flexible definition of women's and men's roles. (Gilbert and Walker 2001)

Seek Input from Your Opposites

There are starters and finishers. There are big-picture people and detail people.

Some people are great at conceiving plans but lose interest in following through on them. And some people are tenacious in seeing a project through but ill suited to dreaming up the next idea. You benefit when you involve people in your projects who have the traits and a perspective that complement your own.

DR. HOWARD MURAD is a Los Angeles–area dermatologist who concluded that many of his patients' concerns about appearance fell at the intersection of medicine and beauty care.

He believed that no one in either business fully appreciated that potential. "I wanted to address the patient's concerns," Dr. Murad explains, "and if that meant using a facialist instead of laser surgery, then that's what I'd do.

"I always ask the question, If you had no disease, would you really be healthy? The answer often is no. What you need to be healthy is a sense of well-being, a sense of the ability to function at your highest level."

Twenty years after merging health and beauty care, Dr. Murad has a $60 million-a-year business selling cosmetic products and spa treatments. But he says none of this would have been possible had he not been "open-minded. I look at things differently, and I bring in people who know things I don't."

Teams in the workplace that are composed of people with differing personalities are 14 percent more productive than teams composed of more similar individuals. (Fisher, Macrosson, and Wong 1998)

Avoid Tanning Beds

Too much exposure to the sun is dangerous and is a leading precursor to skin cancer. However, natural sunlight is far less dangerous than tanning beds.

SHE WAS, BY her own admission, a sun worshipper for most of her life—on the beach all summer, and a regular at tanning beds the rest of the year.

"I was dark. I was very, very dark," says Gayle. "I look back at it now and say, 'How vain.'" The radical change in Gayle's perspective stems directly from a checkup, and the rapid-fire changes it unleashed in her life.

Sitting on an examination table, dressed in a paper gown and awaiting her doctor, Gayle casually asked the nurse what she thought about a mole high on Gayle's right leg. The nurse strongly suggested she show it to the doctor, who, in turn, sent Gayle to see a dermatologist. Immediately.

Gayle had stage-three melanoma, signifying a relatively thick melanoma that had spread to the lymph nodes. Gayle had started down a path that would lead to a pair of surgeries, the removal of fifteen lymph nodes from the right side of her body, and an anguished stretch of time during which she was not sure she would survive.

Fortunately, her disease was caught in time, and doctors have now given her a clean bill of health. "It was just so silly," Gayle says as she relives her days spent in tanning beds. "One thing the cancer has done for me is help me realize the rest of my life will not be devoted to silliness."

Doctors found that tanning beds expose the body to ten to fifteen times higher concentrations of dangerous ultraviolet rays than natural sunlight. (Mount Sinai School of Medicine 2003)

Know What Makes You Happy and What Makes You Sad

Peeople feel worse if they are unhappy but have no idea why. Think about your feelings and emotions. Then, even when you are unhappy, you can take comfort in knowing the cause and how it can be changed.

IT IS NO mystery to Kim why she has felt so lost for many months. In a short time she lost her husband to cancer and her mother to a stroke. But she writes about her life daily in on online journal, in part to give voice to her pain, in part to take special note of the good moments, and in part because it just makes her feel better.

"This is a release for me. I need to rid myself of anger and pain—and I can just put it out there and out of me," Kim says.

Kim writes about everything from the challenge of getting the car repaired to way she feels her identity changing. "You're feeling all these emotions, and nobody seems to understand you," Kim says. "Unless you've been there, you really can't understand."

Kim feels so much love in caring for her children, but at the same time she aches for what she and her children have lost. "Things could be worse," she adds. "We all have tragedy in our lives. I'm charting the good thoughts, the good moments. It's a start, maybe a start toward a good day."

Those who are least likely to quickly overcome a temporary sense of dissatisfaction with life are those who cannot define the sources of their feelings. (Ramanaiah and Detwiler 1997)

Wipe, Don't Blow

Wiping your nose is something you are supposed to outgrow when you are a child. You were probably encouraged from a young age to blow your nose instead. But you should know that there is no scientific reason to avoid wiping your nose and that there are reasons to avoid blowing your nose.

UNIVERSITY OF ARIZONA microbiologist Charles Gerba knows germs. He studies how we spread them to each other and to ourselves.

Handkerchiefs, for example, are an ideal germ spreader. "Organisms persist from one load of laundry to the next, so if you're washing hankies in one load, you're actually blowing your nose on everything you wear, from one load to the next," Dr. Gerba says. Hot water in the laundry will reduce the effect.

But even if you are just blowing your nose into a tissue, "you are spreading virus-laden mucus into the sinuses, causing inflammation," he explains.

Dr. Gerba's advice: "The less dramatic the response, the better." When it comes to your nose, "Let it run, and wipe it on a tissue, and you will not be expending energy to share your germs with others, or to share them with yourself." We need to realize, he says, "that a nose is really a germ cannon, and there are many good reasons to avoid trying to set it off."

Scientists found that the more people with colds blew their nose, the longer their cold lasted. Wiping their nose, on the other hand, caused no worsening of the cold. (University of Virginia 2002)

Do Things in Order

It would be overwhelming, frustrating, and ultimately futile to go after your goals out of order. And yet, we want what we want, and we don't like to wait. Take your goals one at a time, and appreciate the process as you move forward. Otherwise you won't be moving at all.

JAMES MCINTYRE INVESTIGATES airplane crashes. "At an accident, you see where things ended, and then you look backwards to see how they began," James says.

James grew up in poverty in the Bronx, trained to be a pilot in the navy, went to college, and then had a career flying in the navy and for commercial airlines.

He doesn't like to think about his childhood, or his bumpy ride out of poverty, very often.

"Growing up in Fort Apache, I couldn't even imagine this life I've led," James says. "I had to live for the day, because I didn't see much in tomorrow. The navy brought me out of there and paid for college, but before I could think about the future, I had years of service obligated to them. The key for me was to do what I was doing well, and not worry about what would come later. I knew that if I had proper training, I would be in great shape for the rest of my life."

Seven out of ten people who are satisfied with their careers express a strong sense of order—an appreciation for the different phases of a career and their progression to this point. (Elliott 1999)

Avoid Internet Takeover

People have a confusing relationship with the Internet. We very much like to log on and twirl around the Web, check our email, and instant message with friends. But when we shut our computer down, we often feel that we wasted too much time online. The reason is that Internet use for short periods is a mood stimulant, but for long periods it is actually a mood depressant. Psychologists advise that you decide how much time you are going to spend using the Internet before you log on.

MARESSA ORZACK DIRECTS the Computer Addiction Studies Center. When Dr. Orzack began looking into excessive computer use, her colleagues thought she was "totally off the wall," she says. But now she's "swamped" with work. People contact her, by email of course, concerned that their use of the Internet and computers is taking over their life.

Dr. Orzack's early awareness of the problem started at home. "I would sometimes play an online card game so late that I would fall asleep in my chair," she admits.

Dr. Orzack sees people of all ages who lose track of themselves online. "On the surface, a computer game may seem completely harmless. Sending an instant message may seem harmless." she says. "But when it becomes a substitution for life, for human contact, then you have to look at it from a different perspective.

"What's so attractive about going online is that the problems of real life go away for a moment. But, of course, it doesn't solve those problems. In fact, if the Internet is consuming great quantities of time then that is creating new problems for people."

Recurring long periods of personal Internet use were associated with 28 percent lower life satisfaction. (Green et al. 2005)

You Can Worry Your Health Away

Not only are feeling out of control, feeling a sense of dread, and feeling a sense of inadequacy threats to your disposition; they are threats to your health habits. When we feel more vulnerable, we are less likely to maintain healthy habits. We turn to unhealthy and excessive behaviors as a comfort to our feelings, but the relief is quite temporary, while the health effects are lasting.

"STRESS HELPS ACCOUNT for two-thirds of family doctor visits and, according to the U.S. Centers for Disease Control and Prevention, half the deaths of Americans under sixty-five. It has been implicated in heart, stomach, and mental disorders, along with the more ordinary headaches, backaches, and high blood pressure and cholesterol. My study of medical students found decreased levels of the body's natural killer cells, which fight infections and tumors, during stressful times such as exam periods," says Dr. Janice Kiecolt-Glaser of Ohio State University.

Among hormones instrumental in the stress response are adrenaline and cortisol. Although they are energy boosters, they are also potent inhibitors of our immune system. Dr. Kiecolt-Glaser says, "This constant activation of the fight-or-flight response causes various systems of the body to develop chronic problems, such as high blood pressure or a strained heart."

Among Dr. Kiecolt-Glaser's medical students, the ones who diligently practiced relaxation techniques during exam weeks "showed significantly better immune function during exams" than those who did not, she says.

Doctors found that people who experienced high levels of anxiety were up to seven times more likely to practice poor health habits. (University of California, Irvine 2002)

Seek Harmony in Your Life

If part of our life is not working for us, then we will carry that pain into everything else we do. A satisfying life is not one where you feel good about one part of your life and ignore the other parts, but one in which you feel rewarded in everything you care about.

ACTRESS SONDRA LOCKE starred in *The Heart Is a Lonely Hunter,* for which she was nominated for an Oscar. Then she appeared in a series of films starring Clint Eastwood.

A romance began with the first picture they worked on together. "He was more than handsome," she says. "He was compelling. In spite of all the usual bustle and chaos on a movie set, there was a hushed aura surrounding him, like the quiet at the center of a storm."

He invited her to dinner. She accepted. They became inseparable. He bought them a wonderful country property in northern California.

Eastwood frowned on Sondra's interest in expanding her acting career outside his movies. She let her career go—at first only appearing in his movies, and then not appearing in any movies at all.

"I let the relationship be a substitute for my career," Sondra says. "But I didn't realize how much relationships here are more about business than anything else. People in Hollywood on that level—such a high-stakes level—these people make it their business to know the people who will possibly benefit them. As opposed to having a heart connection, a soul connection."

Researchers find a spillover effect such that people who experience high levels of conflict in their relationship are 20 percent less satisfied with their job, and people who experience high levels of stress on the job are 38 percent less satisfied with their personal lives. (Ludlow and Alvarez-Salvat 2001)

Take Small Victories

It may be a long time before you reach your destination. In the meantime, you will need indicators that you are capable, that you are doing the right thing, that eventually you will get where you want to go. Use your small successes to help fuel your journey to your ultimate goal.

LOUIS MINELLA SPENT a career planning every detail of the presentation of department stores. He knew everything about the business of catching the customer's eye and using the layout to maximize sales.

After thirty-one years in the business, he took early retirement. And then he looked for something worthwhile to do.

Louis decided to open a mailing center, where people can ship packages, buy boxes, make copies, and send faxes.

It was a major adjustment. "Instead of being one member of the team in an international organization, I'm in charge of everything," Louis says.

The hands-on difference was most significant: "I was dealing with group managers, regional managers, store managers. I'm in reality now. I used to issue reports and orders, but I didn't personally do the work, or do anything other than tell other people what to do."

He takes great joy from the daily hurdles overcome, like adjusting the hours of his star sixty-six-year-old employee to keep her content, or fixing the leaking ink in the postage meter machine, or figuring out how to copy a seven-hundred-page document.

"It's a different ball game here, but it's tremendously satisfying to learn every little thing that your business needs," Louis says.

Life satisfaction is 22 percent more likely for those with a steady stream of minor accomplishments than for those who express interest only in major accomplishments. (Orlick 1998)

There's Never Been a Better Time

It may not be in the headlines or on the news—but people have never had as long a life expectancy as they do now, and they have never had the capacity to live with health and vigor as long as they do now. Objectively, there has never been a better time to be alive.

HIGH SCHOOL STUDENTS in Bergen County, New Jersey, have a unique opportunity to see the health-care process from the inside. The students shadow workers at Chilton Memorial Hospital, watching everything from the initial care of a newborn to the respiratory tests of a senior citizen.

Students even have the chance to practice some medical procedures —such as trying to insert tubes into a medical mannequin or giving each other stress tests on a treadmill.

"It is amazing what they can do here. It really makes me excited about the opportunities. A nurse's skills are valuable anywhere I might want to go, and would give me a career that helps people," says Shannon, one of the students.

"There have been revolutions in health-care possibilities just in the span of my career," says Elizabeth, a nurse who works with the students during their visits. "And the breakthroughs that are coming are probably beyond my imagination."

Surveys show that 68 percent of people think life is getting harder over time. But anthropologists have found that there has never been a time when we could expect to live as long and be as healthy as we can today. (Veenhoven 2005)

Effort Does Not Equal Success

Work hard and you will be rewarded. It sounds simple. But remember what it was like studying for a test? Some kids studied forever and did poorly. Some studied hardly at all and made great grades. You can spend incredible effort inefficiently and gain nothing. Or you can spend modest efforts efficiently and be rewarded. The purpose of what you do is to make progress, not just to expend yourself.

ACHENBACH'S PASTRIES WAS a Lancaster County, Pennsylvania, institution. The family-owned bakery had a loyal customer base, and had operated profitably for more than four decades.

In the 1990s, the owners decided to expand—to offer deli sandwiches and other goods, and to add new locations for both retail and wholesale.

The bakery's owners had never worked harder in their lives than they did after the expansion. And in return for their hard work, not only were they making less money, but their business was in danger of going bankrupt because they could not keep up with the debts incurred in the expansion.

Earl Hess looked at things as an objective observer and found that the bakery was doomed by inefficiencies. "They had too many products. Ninety percent of sales came from 10 percent of the products. They were losing their aprons making low-volume items," he says.

Hess bought the company, he says, because he realized that the former owners "couldn't possibly have worked any harder, but they could have worked smarter."

Effort is the single most overrated trait in producing success. People rank it as the best predictor of success, when in reality it is one of the least significant factors. Inefficient effort is a tremendous source of discouragement, leaving people to conclude that they can never succeed because they see no results even when they expend maximum effort. (Scherneck 1998)

It's OK to Be Right
When Everyone Else Is Wrong

Responsibility carries with it a special burden. It's not easy to see things differently and to propose what you think is a good path in the face of what might be the popular path. But the long-term importance of making the right decision is far greater than the short-term value of making the pleasing decision.

AFTER BEING A star football player in college, Eddie Shannon spent thirty-five years in the classroom and on the sidelines coaching high school football and basketball near where he grew up on the west coast of Florida.

The father of four and the coach of thousands more, Shannon took that responsibility seriously. "They're all mine. They belong to all of us who care," he says.

Coach Shannon guided his teams to great athletic heights, winning championships in both sports and becoming so successful that other schools avoided scheduling Eddie's teams. His teams were noted for discipline and ferocity.

Coach Shannon was not content with teaching the techniques of sports. He made sure his players were upstanding members of the community. He imposed a 10 o'clock curfew on his players and checked up on them to see that they respected it. His strict style was appreciated by parents, although many students resented the coach's rules.

At a reunion celebrating their coach's lifetime of service, though, former players, ranging from their twenties to their fifties thanked him for instilling the integrity and discipline they continue to live by today.

The responses of children as they age from school age to adult shows that their feelings for their parents and family change, and that more than half feel more positive about their upbringing as they age. (Dorfman 2001)

Think in Concrete Terms

We need to be able to measure our progress, to know that things are improving. You can't accomplish an abstract goal, because you will never be sure if you're finished or not.

DAN IS THE first to admit that what he does is not glamorous. "Nobody will think this is exciting work, but it's important work, and it can mean keeping our people in one piece," Dan says of his job as a safety coordinator for a utility company. Dan's responsibility is to make the company's employees safe on the job, whether they're climbing a utility pole or sitting behind a desk.

"We have a goal—zero accidents and zero incidents. That's the easiest thing to say, but then what do you do with it?" Dan notes. Dan says that a lip-service commitment to safety is a significant danger because, without any meaningful action to make or keep that a reality, it gives people a false impression that things are safe.

Dan takes his message to managers throughout the company with a call for action. "Each of you is accountable for assessing the situation in your area," he tells them. "This means physical inspections, a thorough understanding of any past accidents, and continued communication in both directions between you and every person in your area."

Every step of the way, Dan works on what he calls "the safety model." He says, "You need to see the entire picture—from communication, to action, to result—to keep people properly interested in what you're doing. If we do this right, we do a lot of good for people, and we can build on our own success."

Perceptions that life is meaningful and therefore worthwhile increase 16 percent with concrete thinking. (Lindeman and Verkasalo 1996)

Slow Music for Dinner

We get into routines of food consumption for all kinds of reasons, such as convenience and comfort, that have nothing to do with our biological need for food. Strategies are available to reduce your inclination to overeat that have nothing to do with depriving yourself of the food you need. Listen to slow music while eating, for example, and you will slow yourself down and wind up eating less.

MICHAEL SUFFERED FROM weight and health problems throughout his childhood. Now he runs a fitness camp for children in New England. He knows that kids feel like they are being sent off to prison when they arrive. "They think this is going to be bread and water and lockdowns," he says.

Instead, Michael emphasizes the need for realistic changes, including smaller portions, better nutrition, and more activity. "The campers are so busy with skating, climbing, paddleboats, that they seldom think about food during the day. They realize they are having fun here, and that they are safe here because no one will make fun of them."

To keep the intensity just right, Michael also relies on music: "Music sets the tempo for what we are doing. During activity times, we turn up the fast-paced music the children like to hear. During dinnertime, we have something slower that I like to hear. We tend to mimic the pace of the music we listen to, so the fast music encourages activity, while the slow music helps to encourage a more patient approach to eating."

Researchers found that music can help or hurt dieters. Their study found that the average diner eats five mouthfuls a minute when listening to music with a lively beat, four mouthfuls a minute when listening to no music, and three mouthfuls a minute when listening to a slow melody. (Johns Hopkins University 1997)

A Relationship Requires Two Equals

Relationships crumble under the weight of imbalance. Neither person can be more important. Neither person can be more involved or committed. Neither person can make all the decisions. Neither person can make all the sacrifices. No one gets top billing, because without two equals, there is no relationship.

HE'S AN ATTORNEY. She owns a real-estate firm. They viewed each other as equals in every respect. But even by Trevor's accounting, Susan was handling about 60 percent of the household workload.

Then Trevor handled a case that put things in perspective. "A factory had a two-tracked system for hiring," he recalls. "Men automatically went into a higher-paying scale that had somewhat more variety in the work. Women automatically went into a lower-paying scale where their job was exactly the same every day." After taking the case on behalf of a group of women who argued that this system discriminated against them, Trevor couldn't help but reexamine his home life.

"If our daughter gets sick or the car needs service, it's Susan's day that gets sacrificed. I saw there's no more justification for automatically making Susan handle this than for automatically assigning those women different jobs in the factory," Trevor says.

Trevor's reexamination brought with it a new system where Susan and Trevor rotate duties that disrupt their days, and where Trevor has accepted a number of new household chores. "And we say 'Thank you' and 'You're welcome' instead of arguing about the dishes," Susan says.

The relationships of partners who characterize each other as equal with respect to who makes decisions, who makes sacrifices for the relationship, and who performs household chores are likely to last more than twice as long as relationships where these roles are not shared equally. (Gilbert and Walker 2001)

Cleaning Isn't Clean

Even though the point of cleaning your house is to make it cleaner, the process of cleaning your house actually makes things worse. Cleaning stirs up dust, hair, dander, and other powerful allergens. Ironically, those who schedule their big cleaning of the year to coincide with the arrival of spring are leaving themselves doubly vulnerable, because they will increase the spread of allergens inside their houses just when the amount of allergens outside their houses is peaking.

"I DON'T KNOW anybody who enjoys vacuuming," Carla says. "It's not fun to begin with. Then, it stirs up so much in the air that I can't stop sneezing."

The solution for Carla was a robot.

"Robots are not just for the Jetsons anymore," Carla says. Robots can vacuum your house or mow your lawn, among other sneeze-inducing tasks. "It's good for people who are short on time, elderly people, lazy people, people with handicaps, and allergy sufferers," she adds.

The robot scans the size of the room and then automatically covers the space without any human input. "It may not look like the robots in the movies," she says of the machine that looks like a large radio on wheels. "But this one is real, and it saves time, trouble, and my nose." Carla happily adds, "I let it do its work, and then I enjoy the clean floor."

For most people, allergies can interfere with many aspects of the quality of life, including getting a good night's sleep (68 percent), engaging in outdoor activities (53 percent), being able to concentrate (50 percent), and being productive at work (43 percent). Four out of five people with allergies experience heightened symptoms when cleaning the house. (American College of Allergy, Asthma and Immunology 2002)

Get Experience Any Way You Can

Take the first chance you have to get into the field of your dreams. Even if the job itself is not what you want, you will get a better idea of what that line of work entails, and you will begin to prepare yourself for the job you ultimately desire. On the other hand, you might find out it's not the right job for you and that your future plans need to be adjusted.

FRED MARZOCCHI GREW up with dreams of drawing for a living.

"There aren't many ways to make a living with your sketchbook, but advertising was one of them."

When he couldn't find a job as a commercial artist, Fred became desperate for experience. He found a large drugstore chain with an in-house advertising unit, and literally offered to work for nothing. They took him up on the offer, and within weeks, not only had he gained professional experience, but the drugstore decided to pay him for his efforts.

After working for a number of advertising agencies, Fred went on to open his own graphic-design and photography business. He often looks back on the offer to work without pay. "I just needed a chance, a start in this business, and I haven't had to work for free since," he says with a smile.

College students who served in internships were 15 percent more likely to find employment after graduation, and 70 percent believed they were better prepared for the workplace because of their internship experience. (Knouse, Tanner, and Harris 1999)

Cultivate a Common Interest

Everyone wants to be a positive part of their partner's life and have their partner be a positive part of their life. Much of our days are shut off to that goal as we pursue careers and obligations. That's why it is so important that people look for, or develop, common interests in their relationships. Common interests encourage positive communication and fun and strengthen the sense of connection between partners.

BERT AND DIANE'S idea of fun is to hop into their canoe and paddle the day away together. The Minnesota couple, married more than three decades, decided to take it a little further, though, and planned a four-month journey through the waters and wilderness on the U.S.–Canada border.

"We both love the boundary waters," says Bert. "It's so incredibly beautiful. The trees, the rocks, and the loons. The smell of the pines. The solitude. And us being together. The beauty is enhanced for us because it takes some effort to get there. We love to paddle in the wilderness."

For their journey there were no time schedules and no deadlines. "We're in no hurry to get back to the pressures of everyday life, the world can go on without us knowing about it," Diane explains.

What do they do with all their time out on the water by day and camping on the water's edge by night? "We talk, or there are times when we don't do a lot of talking, which is fine," says Bert.

As for a downside to their common passion? "Mosquitoes. Definitely mosquitoes," he says.

In a comparison of couples who remained together more than five years with couples who split up, researchers found that the couples who stayed together were 64 percent more likely to be able to identify interests that they shared. (Bachand and Caron 2001)

Health Is Mental and Physical

The maximum enjoyment of life follows the pursuit of the care and feeding of both your body and your mind. Symptoms of distress in your life need to be understood in the context of your entire body, not just the immediate area affected. Think of health as a broad goal for both your body and your mind.

IN THE GOLF world, it is known as the yips. The muscles of the hands and wrists spontaneously contract, making it nearly impossible to putt. What was supposed to be an easy three-foot putt can end up feeling like a fifteen-foot putt when a golfer loses control because of the yips. The famous golfer Ben Hogan was afflicted with the yips, and the condition would end his career in professional golf.

"For many years the yips was seen as a purely psychological problem, something that was all in the golfer's head," says Dr. Aynsley Smith of the Mayo Clinic Sports Medicine Center. "We've found that there is both a physical component and mental component to most 'yippers.'"

Mayo Clinic researchers are staging a putting tournament of their own with yippers, including some whose symptoms seem primarily physical and some whose symptoms seem primarily mental. By measuring factors such as confidence, heart rate, grip force, and stress hormones, and by studying the videotapes of each putt, they hope to better understand the problem and offer the best physical and mental treatments to relieve the symptoms.

Doctors found that patients with a physical ailment who received a combination of physical and mental therapies were two and a half times more likely to maintain a long-term successful recovery than patients who received treatment only for their physical condition. (Duke University 2002)

Embrace Challenges

There are many things we wish to do—from changing a tire to changing our lives—that we avoid because we are afraid of failure. We fear the direct evidence of our weakness, so we don't even bother to try. But you are stronger and more capable than you can possibly know.

STARTING WHEN HE was a boy, Sydney Besthoff worked in almost every job in his family's drugstore business until he was eventually promoted to run it. Under his leadership, he helped create one of the largest drugstore chains in the United States.

But after more than fifteen years of running the company, everything Sydney had ever done came under attack. Family members sued him, claiming he had cheated them out of their share of the company's profits.

"It was a cataclysmic blow to him," his wife, Walda, says. "It was heartbreaking for him. He felt betrayed. He was betrayed."

But Sydney did not crumble under the strain of legal action and the animosity of his loved ones. He explained that his strategy of focusing on growth ahead of profits was necessary until the company was big enough to compete with the major chains. "I told them to wait, that they would be very pleased in the end," he says.

Instead, Sydney paid his relatives for their shares of the business. "Anyone else might have folded, lost everything. Sydney found the strength to keep on going. Always rational, even in the face of daunting challenges," Walda says. And in the end, the company continued expanding and succeeding until it was sold to a larger rival chain.

Studies of people who were victims of traumatic events—such as natural disasters that destroyed their homes—found that those people who suffered the most loss of comfort were actually calmer and more resolute than the people who had suffered inconvenience but minimal loss. (Ikeuchi and Fujihara 2000)

Look Up, Literally

Though it may be useful to avoid stepping in things, regularly looking down actually affects our mood. When we look down, we are in a defensive orientation that reinforces a feeling that bad things are likely to happen.

IF YOU WANT to earn a spot on the lifeguard squad in Wrightsville Beach, North Carolina, you have to start with a race against your competitors and the elements. Prospective lifeguards run a mile, then swim half a mile, then swim out and back in two simulated rescues.

"You might think it looks easy, but it's a real challenge, especially when the ocean's not cooperating," says Bud, the chief lifeguard. Applicants are judged by their time and by their ability to properly respond to rescue situations.

The lifeguard competition often attracts people with medical backgrounds, including paramedics. "It's a chance to help people, and it doesn't take place in the back of an ambulance or in an emergency room. It's on the sand and on the water," Bud says.

"This is a job about looking out and looking up. You never stop watching, because you never know when the crucial moment will come," Bud adds. Even if he doesn't have to stir from his guard's chair all day, he says, "I just feel good when I'm out here. I feel more alive."

Looking up as you walk increases the likelihood of being in a good mood by 11 percent. (Meier 2005)

Tell Your Family Story

Caring can come only with knowledge, with a foundation of information that allows one to feel a connection. When we share family history, we strengthen the bond between our family members, and that bond strengthens each individual within the family.

"I'M ONLY TWO generations removed from slavery," says Harold, a lifetime resident of Tennessee. "My great-grandfather was born into slavery until he was nine years old, when the Emancipation Proclamation was passed."

Harold's great-grandfather lived ninety-seven more years after Emancipation. "I listened to a lifetime of his stories. Although after he turned one hundred, the details started getting pretty hazy," Harold says.

Harold, now retired, loves to sit with his grandchildren and tell them his story, and all the family stories he knows dating back to his great-grandfather's childhood. "Look around today. With television, video games, and all that stuff, children hardly know where they came from. Everything looks the same in every town. But if they don't know where they came from, how can they know who they are?" he asks.

Sometimes they roll their eyes or complain they've heard the story before. But Harold mixes in a few adventures with snakes and storms and other scary things, and he brings back their attention. "History is always important. But this is their history. It's their story. And I want to share it so they know it and will tell it to their children one day," Harold says. "I tell them that if you lose this, you can lose it forever. You should know who you are and be proud of who you are wherever you go from here."

Parents who frequently share stories of family history with their children produce higher levels of interest in and concern for family members and increase the likelihood of their children's happiness as an adult by 5 percent. (Leader 2001)

Self-Motivation Works Once

Declare something. What do you want? Declare that you shall have it. Want to be in better shape? Declare that you shall be. Want to get a better job? Declare that you shall have one. We are comforted, energized, enthused by these declarations. Unfortunately, the effects are temporary. Success comes not from self-motivating tricks and declarations of desired outcomes, but from a steady, informed effort at progress.

WHEN DAVID CYNAR was hit by a car at age fifteen, doctors told him he might lose a leg. He thought his life was ruined.

As he looks back on the incident fifteen years later, David sees that the adversity may have saved his life. At the time he didn't care much about anyone or anything, and he had no motivation in school.

But the accident took away his physical strengths and made him look inward for new hope. "I became humbled at a second chance at life. But getting anywhere from there depended on self-confidence and self-worth," he says.

Rehabilitation led him to study karate, and slowly he regained the use of his leg and transformed himself, not only into an athlete, but into a driven person. "Dedication and commitment have to come from inside you, but once you have them, you can go anywhere," David says. Today, he is a successful salesman, a budding country musician, a black belt in karate, and a volunteer mentor for teens.

"I learned the hard way that positive thoughts and actions mean a healthier, happier, more successful life—and I love to share that with everyone I can," David says.

For nearly nine in ten people, declarations of self-change produce a temporary improvement in self-image, followed, in a few weeks, by disappointment that makes their self-image worse than it was before the declaration. (Polivy and Herman 1999)

There Are No Mind Readers

You want support and comfort because of a trying situation. You want your partner to understand the difficulty you face and to make you feel better—even if you don't actually say these things or explain the situation. We often set our partners up to fail us in these situations by not fully disclosing our feelings and the situation as we perceive it. When you need support, say so.

ED WORKS IN a California-based public-relations firm. His boss is his wife, Gwen.

"For spousal business relationships to work requires mutual admiration," Ed says. "I have a lot of respect for Gwen and her abilities. If she were less proficient, I probably wouldn't have come to work for her.

"You have to be pretty secure in your masculinity, though," he continues. "But Gwen is a genius, and I think I'm good at what I do."

Gwen is also admiring of her husband's skills. "He could sell ice to Eskimos," she says.

Despite all their mutual respect, problems inevitably arise. "Ed will get so wrapped up in making sure everything runs right that he will turn and give me a direction like he's talking to an employee," Gwen says. "That irritates me."

But Gwen doesn't hide irritation from Ed. Nor does Ed shy away from noting when he feels Gwen is bringing her office role home.

Such circumstances are inevitable and highlight the need for open communication to head off extreme conflict. "We have to say what we mean—with no underlying messages," says Ed. "If the emotional message is different from the content, that's a problem."

Researchers found that those who are more direct in seeking support from their partner are 61 percent more likely to feel they received the support they wanted. (Fitness 2001)

Do What You Say You Are Going to Do

Nothing kills progress or deadens enthusiasm more than someone who talks but never follows through. It is crucial in both your home life and your work life that you stay focused and committed to whatever you say you will do.

BOB WAS LOOKING for a new line of work. Already past the age when most people retire, he knew that some would think he was too old to learn anything new.

But Bob had always been fascinated by planes, and one day he just presented himself at the small airport near his home outside Memphis. He didn't know much about planes, but Bob's background as a former marine convinced the general manager that Bob could be counted on. Bob's tasks include fueling aircraft, which sometimes means climbing up on their wings. But without him literally nothing can happen at the airport.

Bob's boss says he hired him because he had "something we see in very few workers: ethics. I had somebody that I knew would be here when we needed him."

As Bob says, "There is no 'almost' in aviation. This is a job for getting things done."

People who have a high rate of following through on their commitments are 41 percent more likely to express confidence in themselves and 28 percent more likely to say they feel in control of their lives. (Stewart, Carson, and Cardy 1996)

Put Stuff in Its Place

Understand the limited value of the things you can buy. The pursuit of all things bigger and newer drives people to jump on an unfulfilling treadmill of getting money and spending money. Define the things you truly value, but do not let yourself get caught buying for the sake of buying.

PAM HELPS PEOPLE organize their stuff. "People get too much stuff, and it starts to take over their homes," she says. Pam changes the layout of closets, helps consolidate things, and ultimately tries to get the owner to consider how much of what they have is really necessary. "Then, after I'm done, if I've done a good job, their home functions better and stuff won't overwhelm them," Pam says.

Her theory is that clutter drains energy and creativity, and that getting rid of it opens the door to greater productivity, personal growth, and peace.

It was a sad irony for Pam when her aunt died and Pam inherited her aunt's home. "It was packed with things in no discernable order," she recalls. "There were valuable items mixed in with things that were sentimentally valuable mixed in with things that seemed to have no purpose whatsoever."

Pam encourages people to think through what they have and what they value, especially items of personal and family significance. "People think they will have endless time to sort through things and make sense of it all. But it slips down on the list, and if they don't act, many unique and personally treasured items get lost in the crowd," Pam says.

People for whom materialism was the main priority had the lowest life satisfaction. (Ryan and Dziurawiec 2001)

History Isn't Everything

For many diseases, a family history is a risk factor for you in getting the disease. But that does not mean you are likely to get the disease or that you are powerless to improve your chances of avoiding the disease. Knowing your family history should help you be better informed about potential risks, but it should not be a source of alarm.

FOR KATE, IT started with a health assignment her son received in school. "He was supposed to create a family tree, but with health information included. Four generations of mental and physical ailments," she says.

Kate soon found out how difficult it can be to assemble such information. "I had most of the information for my parents, my aunt and uncle, but I had trouble with my grandparents, and my great-grandparents were people I had never met. My husband's side of the family is big and spread out across the country," she says.

Spurred on originally by an interest in helping her son with the assignment, Kate became engrossed in the investigation. "It was like police work—tracking people down, putting the information together," Kate says. "I really became fascinated with the information and its implications for myself, my husband, and my son."

Several weeks later, her son had finished the family tree. It lists predispositions, disease frequency, and the potential for everything from hypertension to depression.

Kate understands both the power and the limits of this information: "Too many people discover their family medical history only after disaster has struck in the form of cancer or other heartbreaking diseases. But this is not a call to panic. It is a call to prepare and empower, to remove fear from this process, and to understand our vulnerability."

Only 5 percent of cancer diagnoses are considered to have hereditary origins. (Mayo Clinic 2002b)

There's No Point to Putting on a Show

There are many people who are content but unhappy. They are unsatisfied with their relationship, but they have little inclination to end it. Why? They seek the presentation value to family and friends of being in a relationship. But there is no satisfaction and no fulfillment in being in a relationship that does not meet your needs.

WHEN KELLY RUTHERFORD, an actress who starred on *Melrose Place*, married Carlos Tarajano, a bank executive, in Beverly Hills, the scene was memorable. Kelly wore a Carolina Herrera gown and toted a three-carat-emerald-encrusted ring on her finger. Guests celebrated in the Sunset Room of the Beverly Hills Hotel late into the night. It was such an event that *InStyle* magazine profiled the spectacular ceremony in its February 2002 issue.

By the time the issue hit the newsstands, filled with dazzling pictures of the happy couple, Kelly Rutherford had filed for divorce.

The magazine has also published features on the weddings of comedian Tom Green to actress Drew Barrymore and of actress Courtney Thorne-Smith to Andrew Conrad after the paperwork had been filed for dissolutions. The marriage of actress Helen Hunt to actor Hank Azaria and of Jennifer Lopez to Ojani Noa survived past publication date but ended within weeks of being profiled.

Sociologist David Blankenhorn says that this strange pattern is in part a reflection of trends in society as a whole. "When marriage is a show, it's prone to being cancelled," he says. "We need, as a society, to pay less attention to the appearance of our relationships and more attention to their reality."

One in five married persons reported that they found their relationship unsatisfying but did not wish to make any changes because they were aware of the status value of being married. (Nock 2001)

Speak Slowly

We have a lot to say, and only a short time to say it in. The natural tendency is to try to pack as much in as we can. But communication is not about the number of things we say, it's about the number of things that are understood. Good speakers master a practice that is simple but powerful: they speak more slowly than others.

NEWSMAN DAVID BRINKLEY'S distinctive delivery is known to generations.

He was a pioneer in network news, first anchoring the original NBC news report, then going on to host the Sunday-morning news-analysis program *This Week.*

He credits a teacher's simple advice for a great deal of his success: "He said to me, 'The faster you speak, the less people will understand you. Take that to heart.' And I did."

People rate speakers who speak more slowly as being 38 percent more knowledgeable than speakers who speak more quickly. (Peterson, Cannito, and Brown 1995)

Pursue What You Need Forever, Not What You Want Today

We are happy when we get what we want. Aren't we? Actually we are happy when we get what we want only if what we want serves our needs. Getting exactly what we want at any given minute would be the same as a child getting candy for every meal. While happy when first given the candy, he will over time grow tired of candy and have rotten teeth. View the search for a happy relationship not as a process of immediate satisfaction but as a means to pursue your fundamental needs.

BRENDA AND MARTY are dedicated to each other and to the children they serve in state-run children's services agencies. Unfortunately, they work for different states.

They can't see each other every day, but they email each other several times a day. "We write about our days, our work, our dogs," says Brenda.

Brenda and Marty do spend every other weekend together. "The weekends we're together are like honeymoons. We spend lots of time doing fun things. I think most married folks don't devote two entire weekends a month to their relationships like we do," Brenda says

"But this life is not for everyone," Marty says. "You have to believe and trust your partner. You have to spend quality, nurturing, and loving time together. I think a lot of marriages don't work because living together on a daily basis is very difficult. We appreciate each other more because of the time we spend apart."

Couples who pursue a hedonistic form of happiness, seeking to fulfill their desires regardless of consequences, endure twice as much conflict as couples who pursue more altruistic forms of happiness—that is, happiness based on creating feelings of unity and mutual satisfaction. (Loveless 2000)

Don't Buy the Fountain of Youth

The claims are tempting. Look younger! Feel younger! Reverse the effects of aging! And get all that in a pill or a cream. These are claims with no basis in reality, however. You cannot buy youth. In fact, not only will you waste your money, but you might do yourself harm in the process. Instead, focus your energy on habits and behaviors that reduce the effects of aging.

THE SIMPLE FACT is that "no currently marketed intervention has yet been proved to slow, stop, or reverse human aging," says Dr. Jay Olshansky of the University of Illinois at Chicago.

Dr. Olshansky regularly makes announcements highlighting antiaging products that he says make outrageous claims. One such product touts its use by Princess Caroline, John Wayne, Yul Brynner, Anthony Quinn, Natalie Wood, and many other worldwide dignitaries, including members of the KGB before Communism fell. As Dr. Olshansky notes, "Ironically, not only is the inventor of the product dead, so are many of the people he brags about having used his product.

"This is just one of many products being sold throughout the world with the claim that they will slow or reverse human aging," Dr. Olshansky continues. "These products have never been proven to do anything but line the pockets of those selling them.

"Although there is reason to be optimistic that scientists will eventually be able to intervene in one or more processes associated with human aging," Dr. Olshansky warns, "it is not currently possible to buy a product that will stop or reverse aging."

Americans spend more than $15 billion on antiaging products every year. None have been subject to government testing, and a majority are considered potentially harmful by government doctors. (University of Illinois at Chicago 2003)

Make Your Mark on the Next Generation

We need to know that we accomplished something. We need to know that what we did had some lasting value. There is no better way to meet those goals than to influence the next generation. Whether it is through family, a friendship, or a community group, or even if our goal is to benefit people we'll never know, we need to see that what we've done continues. Keep the next generation in the forefront of your goals, and you will feel the benefits of their future.

RITA DIDN'T HAVE a lot. She didn't have a lot of money, and she didn't have a lot of free time. But the time Rita did have she loved to spend in her garden. Rita planted almost every inch of her backyard with vegetables. Every day before and after work her neighbors would see her out back, wearing her boots, weeding, planting, watering, and caring for her tomatoes, corn, squash, carrots, and cucumbers.

But it's what she did with her vegetables that impressed her neighbors most. Living in a poverty-stricken area, Rita was not only willing to share what she had, but insisted that her neighbors share in the bounty. And for those who had no idea what to do with a squash, Rita was ready with recipes and ideas.

Health problems eventually slowed Rita down and kept her from her garden. Instead of missing the season, though, her neighbors planted it for her. "I swear, the only reason half the children in the neighborhood ever saw a fresh vegetable was because of Rita," one neighbor says. "You don't meet too many inspirational people, but Rita is an inspiration."

If you know someone's age, income, and health you are four times less likely to successfully predict whether they are happy than if you know whether they can identify a positive effect they are having on a younger person. (Azarow 2003)

Do One Thing at a Time

W hen there are a lot of things we should be doing, we want to take on as many tasks as possible. But trying to do all those things at one time will ensure only that we accomplish none of them.

ACTOR LUIS GUZMAN has appeared in films such as *Traffic* and *Magnolia* and on television dramas including *Oz, NYPD Blue,* and *Law & Order* and has starred in a television comedy, *Luis,* named for him.

With a busy professional life, Luis has an even busier personal life. He and his wife are parents of four adopted children.

Luis wanted his family to enjoy a life as free as possible from the pressures and distractions most actors endure. So he left the big city and took his family to Vermont.

"I wanted my kids to be able to come out of their door and get on their bikes and walk around. A place where I don't have to worry about them," Luis says. "I wanted them to grow up in a place where people know each other. And where the last thing on my mind would be work. I just made the conscious choice that this is where I wanted to raise my family so I can have the focus of family and not have the distractions of the city."

Even in Vermont, though, Luis admits, he can't completely get away from his job: "It's a small town and it's like 'Wow, we know somebody on a TV show and he lives next door. Let's take him some corn.'"

People who carried worries about their family to their work, or worries about their work to their family, were 32 percent less likely to be satisfied with their lives and 44 percent more likely to feel out of control than people who segmented their thinking by keeping their work and family concerns separate. (Sumer and Knight 2001)

Remember Who You Are and Where You Are

A big organization, by definition, must ask its people to put their own individuality aside and work as a group. If you work for a big organization, there is little room for some of the aspects of your life that are most central to you, be they religious beliefs or cultural traditions. Those who express satisfaction with their accomplishments know that they can never toss aside the beliefs, customs, and values that they hold dear; they just display them on their own time.

BOBBY RICHARDSON PLAYED second base for the New York Yankees in the 1950s and 1960s.

Bobby went to work in an atmosphere that differed so much from his sheltered religious upbringing that he could hardly describe it to his family back home.

He knew that he had to keep his religion in his life, but he also knew that he couldn't bring it into the locker room or the dugout. That is why he helped found the Baseball Chapel.

Richardson's group met off the field and out of the limelight, and brought together teammates and players from opposing teams, to share their faith.

Bobby explains, "You have to do something to make sure you aren't swallowed whole by the big leagues. But you can't impose who you are on everybody else, so the Baseball Chapel let me be a teammate on company time and be who I really was on my time."

Those who express the most satisfaction with their lives and careers tend to utilize a hybrid view of themselves. They are a combination of the capable, team-oriented person on the job and a culturally and spiritually distinct person at home. Those who sacrifice their individual beliefs and backgrounds ultimately express one-third less satisfaction with their jobs and almost two-thirds less satisfaction with their lives. (Franklin and Mizell 1995)

Relationships Are Not Random

In all aspects of your life, you will feel a greater sense of satisfaction and less stress if you maintain a sense of control. You have to recognize that your decisions shape your life, regardless of what else might be happening around you. A healthy relationship will foster the sense that your decisions matter, while an unhealthy relationship will make you feel that your decisions are irrelevant.

MADGE AND EDDIE have been married for more than seven decades. During their marriage they've seen twelve presidents come and go.

What put so much staying power in their wedding vows? "Love," says Madge. "That's all."

There was, of course, mutual respect and patience. And what Madge calls "a Midwestern mind-set, a sort of stick-to-itiveness common among folks from a certain time."

Eddie says their arguments helped a lot, too—little disagreements, each followed quickly by forgiveness. "We'd get mad. We might not speak to each other. But later that day, you wouldn't know it," says Eddie.

"Well," Madge adds, "he might pout for a while."

For Madge, such marital know-how comes from "good old common sense. You have to give and take. But you've got to keep control of yourself all the time. Never take it too far."

If things were too much for Madge, she took an occasional weekend for herself. "I still like to be alone sometimes," she says. "If you can't stand yourself, how can you stand anybody else?"

But, as Madge is quick to point out, "I'm still in love. I love the old bugger and wouldn't want to get rid of him."

People with a sense of control in their lives, in both career and relationship, were 66 percent more likely to report feeling happy and satisfied. (Chou and Chi 2001)

Emergencies Can't Wait

When an emergency strikes, will you immediately call for help? Although the answer would seem obvious, most people fail to act quickly, and even when they decide to act, they fail to call for help. When emergency situations occur, we must throw out our normal habits of caution and restraint and immediately seek the help of professionals.

THE SINK IN the bathroom was running, and firefighters found a container of water nearby after they dragged the man, unconscious, from an intensely hot and smoky apartment fire in Syracuse, New York.

As stunned neighbors watched, firefighters laid the man on a snowy driveway, pumped his chest, and puffed oxygen into his lungs. The firefighters could not save him.

It appears he tried to douse the flames himself before smoke overwhelmed him, authorities said. He did not dial 911. "People think they can tolerate the smoke conditions because they watch movies like *Backdraft,* which is ridiculous," says Syracuse firefighter Lt. Jeff Sargent.

The fire was so hot that the couches were scorched to their springs and the television melted down to its tube.

"The only message is 'Get out,'" says John Cowin, Syracuse fire chief. "A small fire doubles every minute. This is an unfortunate situation. Whenever you are dealing with a fire emergency, a police emergency, or a medical emergency, call it in immediately. Give us a chance to do our jobs."

Doctors found that nearly half of almost 800,000 heart-attack patients they studied drove themselves or were driven by a friend or family member to the hospital instead of calling 911 for an ambulance. This occurred even though emergency medical personnel can cut in half the time it takes to receive potentially life-saving treatments such as clot-buster drugs. (University of Alabama at Birmingham 2002)

Treat the Disease, Not the Symptom

Disagreements are inevitable. In trying to overcome them, many of us adopt a strategy of attempting to fix the immediate problem at hand. If your partner complains that you don't go out and have fun enough, you plan a big Saturday night out. Generally, though, major complaints present themselves as mere symptoms, not the disease. That is, the problem isn't what you are doing this Saturday night, but a general feeling of boredom. If you address only the immediate symptom, the real problem won't go away.

"IT'S ALMOST TOO dumb to talk about," Sam admits, but his girlfriend Laura was a television vulture. "If you're watching a game, and reading the newspaper at the same time, she'll come in and grab the remote, and the next thing you know Martha Stewart is on, telling us how to make curtains.

"I'll say, 'I was watching that,' and she'll say, 'No, you weren't.' And the next thing you know, it's a big thing."

At a loss as to how to settle their recurring dispute, they finally brought in a trusted third party for some help. "My sister said we're both making me-first assumptions," Sam says. "That I was reading and watching the game as if our whole world revolved around me, and that she was snookering the television remote as if I wasn't there. It is amazing how quickly the petty squabbles go away when you understand the big picture of sharing and caring and really treating each other as you wish to be treated."

Couples who openly share their thoughts and their perspectives related to areas of conflict are 18 percent more likely to report that their disagreements often produce solutions and are 12 percent more likely to say they are satisfied in their relationships. (Palmer-Daley 2001)

Help the Next Person
Who Needs Some Minor Assistance

Giving help is a win-win situation, so take the time to pay attention to your surroundings and offer the help that you can. It could be as simple as holding the door open for the person behind you. It is a gesture of friendliness that makes another person feel better and makes you feel good about yourself.

STACY MOVED TO the Midwest from the Northeast and quickly noticed that people in the Midwest seemed to be in the habit of being courteous drivers. If you were stuck trying to get out of a parking lot, with a mile-long procession of cars in front of you on the main road, people in the Midwest would stop and give you room to pull out.

Based on this example, Stacy got in the habit of letting cars out when traffic was backed up. Stacy liked this friendly approach to life and soon received a dramatic example of its value.

After letting a car out in front of her, Stacy soon had to pull over to the side of the road because her car was making a strange noise. The driver she had let out saw her pull over and followed her. The driver asked Stacy if she needed any help and after a brief investigation concluded that Stacy had just run out of gas. He gave her enough gas to get her to a station and told her how nice he found people in this part of the country. She gave him her telephone number, and one year later they were married.

Life satisfaction was found to improve 24 percent with the one's level of altruistic activity. (Williams, Haber et al. 1998)

Negotiate with Confidence, or Don't

Y ou will face many negotiations in your life—whether for a pay raise or over the terms of a car purchase. Ultimately, your willingness to continue negotiations is based on your own level of self-confidence. No matter what your other advantages might be, you will end negotiations faster if you lack confidence, which means you'll settle for a less advantageous resolution.

ROBERT GOTTLIEB HAS spent a life working with writers, eventually becoming editor of the *New Yorker* after spending a career in publishing. He is noted for being sought out for his critical insights by renowned writers such as Joseph Heller and Toni Morrison.

He has a lifetime of experience negotiating everything about a piece of writing, from the payment to the punctuation. He even told Joseph Heller that "Catch–18" wasn't as good a title as Gottlieb's suggestion, "Catch–22."

His theory of negotiating is simple: "If you're saying, 'Well, I don't know. Maybe. What do you think?' that's not helping. You have to be able to say what you believe, in an unaggressive and uncontentious way. You have to believe it; then, negotiate as if it were true. Whereas if you do not believe yourself, you cannot help. You have to be forceful."

Lower self-worth translates into 37 percent less willingness to negotiate and using 11 percent fewer negotiation strategies. Increased self-worth correlates with greater willingness to incur the risks of prolonged negotiation and greater adaptability. In short, the less confidence you have in yourself, the faster you will give up trying to get what you want. (Greno-Malsch 1998)

Your Surroundings Will Affect Your Health Approach

While we are all capable of making decisions on our own, we often let ourselves be influenced by people around us. If we see our family, friends, and neighbors out taking long walks or jogging, we are more likely to participate. On the other hand, if people around us have unhealthy habits, we are more likely to ignore the importance of health. Pay attention to the good examples around you, and if you don't have any, understand that you will have to set the good example.

THEY USED TO be a family that sat around together. Now, they are a family that exercises together.

Chris and Theresa, forty-something parents of ten-year-old Danny, decided that the family should get out and exercise more. They had very different motivations: Chris was concerned about his overall fitness, Theresa about trying to improve chronic back problems, and Danny felt confined by a school day that contained no recess or gym class. However, they realized they would all do more if they did it together.

They now go to the gym together at least once a week. Chris favors the elliptical trainer, Theresa the weight machines, and Danny does a bit of everything.

"We exercise together all the time," Theresa says. "Alone, I couldn't get motivated to do it. It's easier to back out when no one else is involved. But as a family, it's a family project, it's a team, and the motivation is always there."

People who described their friends and neighbors as having favorable attitudes toward exercise and healthy eating were 19 percent more likely to have healthy exercise and eating habits themselves. (University of Minnesota 2002a)

Money Can't Buy Love, but It Can Buy Stress

What is the single most important part of your life? It's not money. It never has been, and it never will be. But how many times has a disagreement about money—how to spend it, how to get it, how much is enough—gotten in the way of your enjoyment of time with loved ones? Put money in its place—behind what really matters to you.

"THE AVERAGE PERSON abuses money," says Steve Rhode of Myvesta, a financial-counseling program headquartered in Maryland. He talks about abusing money in the same way others might warn of abusing or becoming addicted to a substance. Steve runs a program that incorporates an emphasis on life and relationship skills, because they are nearly inseparable from money use.

Steve warns that what makes our use of money even more dangerous is that this use is often overlooked, treated as a frivolous situation instead of as a problem. "Many people assume that it's normal to be unable to control their money. It's not. People get stuck because they deny that a problem exists, which holds them back from conquering their money issues.

"People conceal their money habits, argue over money habits, let money habits dictate who they are," Steve says. "There is just no way to deny that your money habits will affect your relationship."

Steve's message to clients is to focus on what is truly important to them while monitoring their spending impulses. "We try to fill up holes in our lives by spending money on them," Steve says. "There's no point trying to fill the holes in your life with money, because you can keep pouring cash in them and you will never fill them."

Financial disagreements are a significant source of conflict in more than half of all relationships. Interestingly, this problem occurs regardless of income level. (Goldscheider 2001)

Where You Stand Depends on Where You Look

A re you doing well? Average? Below average? These judgments, in truth, are entirely relative. Feelings of success are based on our position relative to those who've accomplished less. Feelings of failure are based on our position relative to those who've accomplished more. Your feelings are as dependent on your frame of comparison as they are on anything you've done.

TODAY, LIKE ANY other day, Roger was out the door and at his desk by 8 A.M. The Cleveland-area corporate accountant was in his twenty-fourth year with the same company.

By lunchtime, he was called in to the head of the division's office and told that his services were no longer needed.

"When something like this happens, it really shakes you to your core. I don't care how prepared you are," Roger remembers.

The devastation was incredible, and the denial followed. "This couldn't possibly be happening to me," Roger thought.

Roger read articles and books on dealing with layoffs, and found stories of men who were so devastated by what had happened that they continued to dress and leave for work every morning, even though they no longer had a job, because they couldn't face telling their families.

Roger began to see his situation in a different light. He still ached at the rejection, but he realized that he had enjoyed more than two decades of work that had allowed him to prosper and provide for his family.

Doing volunteer fund-raising work made him appreciate his situation all the more. "Think about the folks who have seen nothing but setbacks," Roger says, "and you'll realize all the good that lies ahead."

Excellent students in gifted-student programs are 36 percent less likely to consider themselves "well-above-average students" than are similar students who remain in regular school populations. (Zeidner and Schleyer 1999)

Keep Going

It's hard to get much done one little step at a time. But it's impossible to get anything significant accomplished without going one little step at a time.

JUST OUT OF medical school, Dr. Robert Lopatin was working 100-hour weeks as a first-year medical resident. Unlike other residents, who often drew skeptical looks from patients wondering if they were really old enough to be a doctor, Robert seemed to inspire a calm confidence in patients. In fact, not a single one questioned whether he was old enough be a doctor.

It could have had something to do with the fact that he was fifty-five years old.

As a boy, Robert had imagined himself as a doctor. But when his father asked him for help, Robert dedicated the next three decades to the family business.

When the business was sold to a competitor, however, the newly unemployed Robert knew exactly what he wanted to do with his time.

At age fifty-one he began studying at the Albert Einstein College of Medicine in New York City. He was older than most of his professors. He was even older than the school itself. But he felt completely at ease. "It took a lot of imagination to do it, but it just felt so right," he says.

Dr. Lopatin now practices in New York. And he encourages others to keep going, even if they didn't quite get where they were heading when they were younger. "When you're older, once you do make a commitment to something, there's more purposefulness, and there's more joy," he says.

People in their sixties and beyond who had a long-term plan to accomplish something were 31 percent more likely to report that they enjoyed their lives. (Wallace, Bisconti, and Bergeman 2001)

Overcome the Culture of Failure

We imagine a life in which all accomplishments are valuable and therefore praised. But we live in a world where far too often accomplishments are threatening and discouraged. Classmates, co-workers, supervisors, and even spouses can see unusual accomplishments as a threat to their standing if they see themselves falling behind in comparison. Do not depend on encouragement to achieve what you want.

HIS CLIENT WAS a county prosecutor accused of corruption. The state put its best people on the prosecution team. The original defense attorney dropped out, and that left Ted Wells trying his very first case. In a stunning outcome, his client was acquitted.

Instead of the respect of his colleagues, though, Ted won mostly their skepticism. "I think a lot of people were jealous because it was such an enormous win," says one colleague and friend. "They started to pooh-pooh his performance and said it was luck and it wasn't skill. A lot of people were threatened by Ted."

Ted never let the slights of his colleagues dampen his enthusiasm for the job. "I do what I love to do, which is solve people's problems," he says. "That's what I think I do pretty well."

In fact, he views keeping a level head as a great asset in the courtroom. "Arrogance and lack of compassion come through to a jury, and they do your client no good whatsoever," Ted says.

More than eight in ten people in upper management positions reported that they encountered denigration of the achievements in their lives. (Rundle-Gardiner and Carr 2005)

Play the Odds

There is an element of chance in everything. Every aspect of your education and career has been affected by quirks of fate. New opportunities are seen or missed depending on who is paying attention. Still, you have to embrace the uncertainty of outcomes and realize that chance can play for you or against you on any given day. But the more you try, the greater your opportunity to benefit from a lucky outcome.

REBECCA ADAMS WANTED a challenge, and she wanted to do something for her community. At fifty-seven, she decided she wanted to run for city council in her hometown of Chesapeake, Virginia.

She ran even though local political experts said the political newcomer didn't stand a chance: "Nobody out-and-out said, 'You're too old,' but people said things like 'Is this really what you want to do with your time and energy at this point?' And I said yes.

"We all have the same 10,080 minutes in a week," Rebecca adds. "We can spend them worrying, or we can do something more productive with them."

While she very much wanted to win the election and serve her city, her expectations were modest. There were fifteen candidates for one seat, but though the odds were against her, she knew she couldn't win if she didn't run.

With no experience, little money, but lots of hard work, she won the race. With a seat on the city council, she has her mind firmly focused in one direction. "We've got to decide what we want to look like in the future," Rebecca says, referring both to her hometown and to its people.

Career analysts find that 83 percent of midcareer professionals believe chance played a significant role in their ultimate career path and that they highly value staying open to unexpected opportunities. (Williams, Soeprapto et al. 1998)

Decide Whether You Want to Win or Be Happy

There is only one real question you must face in an argument: Do you want to win by showing how right you are, or do you want to compassionately come to a resolution with your partner? You can win all the arguments you want, and feel good about always being right. But you will not have helped yourself in the slightest. Or you can give up thinking about who won and lost, because in truth, either you both win the argument or you both lose.

COLMAN McCARTHY TEACHES conflict resolution to children and adults. He tells people to approach conflict in a healthy way.

"Define the situation objectively," Colman recommends. "What is the situation, what needs to happen to improve it? This simple step is crucial. Sociologists report that in as many as 75 percent of husband-wife fights, the combatants are battling over different issues. The husband may be enraged over what his wife said or did that morning. The wife is out of control over what her husband did ten weeks ago. They can't settle their conflict because they don't know what it's about."

The next step, Colman says, is to "realize the contest involved. It's not you against me, it's you and me against the problem. By focusing on the problem, and not on the person with the problem, a climate of cooperation, not competition, is enhanced."

Colman admits that sometimes the partners in conflict are so emotionally wounded that nothing can help. "But large numbers of conflicts can be resolved, provided the strategies for peacemaking are known," Colman says. "Gandhi said, 'Don't bring your opponents to their knees, bring them to their senses.'"

People who maintained a compassionate spirit during disagreements with their partner had 34 percent fewer disagreements, and the disagreements they did have lasted 59 percent less time. (Wu 2001)

Travel the Stable Road

You can't have peaks without valleys. It is a simple law of nature. Your emotional highs will give way to emotional lows. The best route to consistently feeling good is to see the value of the plateau.

THE FIRST BASEMAN had cancer. The second baseman, shortstop, and third baseman have all had heart attacks. "And if you think that's bad, wait until you hear about the shape of our outfielders," says Ted.

On this softball team for men in their fifties, sixties, and seventies, major health difficulties have been a part of almost every player's life.

And yet, those problems are rarely discussed. "We don't talk medicine," Ted says. "Very seldom do we talk about ailments and hurts, because we've all had them. So we play through them and don't think about it. We're having fun."

They make an exception for discussing on-field injuries. Ted and his teammates love to talk about the time he tripped while rounding third base and broke his leg. When it happened, the first words he heard from a league official were not "Are you OK?" or "Do you need some help?" Instead, Ted says, "the guy says to me, 'You're out.'"

The bottom line for Ted and his teammates is simple. "We can all still hit. And the rest of the day goes a little smoother after you've knocked one over the right fielder's head," Ted says.

People who experienced fewer dramatic changes in mood were 21 percent more likely to maintain an optimistic outlook on life. (Hills and Argyle 2001)

Mold Is Everywhere—Relax

There are one hundred thousand different kinds of mold. You can find many of them in just about any home. The vast majority of these mold types are harmless, however. Despite the sometimes scary headlines, small amounts of mold in your home don't mean you will wind up with a serious illness. Nor do they mean you have anything to fear.

STEVE MAKES HIS living from mold. His Arkansas company cleans heating and cooling duct systems to remove mold. And business has been booming.

"Every time there's a story on the news about mold in homes, we get ten calls," Steve says.

Steve says he finds mold in every home he visits, but he also admits, "Is it that black deadly mold? I couldn't tell you.

"As long as we have humidity, moisture, and leaks, we're going to have mold problems," he says. "Mold is here to stay."

As for advice, Steve says that households need to think about reducing the likelihood of major mold problems. Repair water leaks promptly, vent bathrooms, and reduce indoor humidity with vents, dehumidifiers, or air conditioners. And though he knows it's not good for business to say so, Steve admits that "people shouldn't be panicking about this."

Most people have no adverse reaction to mold. Scientists have been unable to substantiate reports of mold-induced chronic ailments. (Mayo Clinic 2003)

The Most Time Is Not the Best Time

If we have found the one person in the world we most want to spend our time with, then why not spend as much time as possible with that person? Because relationships thrive on the quality of contact, not the quantity of contact. For most people, a little distance every day is necessary for their own independent interests and needs. Some time apart serves to strengthen the relationship by giving both partners a chance to feel an active need for each other, and to experience the pleasure of reuniting.

CARLA AND BRIAN run a bus line that provides tours of Boston. They divorced after a fifteen-year marriage but continue to amicably operate the business they started together ten years ago.

"When we decided to end the marriage, we did it with a small realization that we had perhaps put more into the business than we had into our marriage," Carla says. "We made a sad but conscious decision to save the business and let the marriage go."

"We all have a tendency when we're under stress and things are not going so well to blame others," Brian says. "It's a particular risk for couples who are in business together. If they're having some sort of problems or challenges in the business, it's just really easy to turn on your spouse and blame each other." He advises couples who work together to develop significant independent activities away from work—and from each other. "What happens for a lot of couples in business is they end up being in each other's space so intensely that between home and work, they can really start to lose perspective."

Seventy-six percent of newly retired married couples say they face a challenge dealing with the greatly increased time spent in each other's company. (Szinovacz and Schaffer 2000)

The Past Is Not the Future

It's tempting to simplify things: "The game is rigged. Some people have all the advantages, and they succeed. Some people have all the disadvantages, and they fail." It is also, however, terribly misleading. Your success is far more dependent upon your behavior now than it is upon where you grew up, where you went to school, whether your path has so far been easy or difficult. Opportunity lies ahead; it's just a matter of whether you choose to pursue it.

JOHN PETERMAN HAD an idea to create a unique retail catalog and transform himself into J. Peterman.

Thirty-five investors in a row told him it was losing proposition.

The thirty-sixth invested $1 million.

His sales philosophy is based on awakening your imagination, because "your imagination is far more powerful than anything I could show you or tell you," John says.

How did he keep going in the face of so many rejections? "You fail a lot in life. Success is just overcoming failures," John answers. He compares the process of moving on after a failure to playing baseball: "If you think about your error, you'll make another error. Making mistakes is just a learning process."

John's start down the road to success began with a childhood lived in modest circumstances. "By today's standards we were poor, but I didn't realize it," he says. Instead, he focused on what he did have. "I had ample opportunity to have nothing to do but have a vivid imagination," he adds.

The current pattern of behavior that employees engage in (both inside and outside the office) is six times more likely to predict job performance than are their background and job history. (Arrison 1998)

Look on the Bright Side

In almost everything that happens, you will have the opportunity to consider the worst or the best implications. Even in terrible setbacks, there are rays of hope you might focus on. And even in wonderful events, there are threads of worry or despair you might cling to. Your focus is not merely a personality quirk, but a way of life. Not only will learning to see the upside, the optimistic outcome, the good in what has happened increase your enjoyment of life; it will lengthen your life.

SHE'S EIGHTY-TWO YEARS old. She has outlived two husbands. But Annie enjoys every day.

"I can do anything I want today," Annie says, and she just might.

"You can close yourself off, say 'Poor me.' But what kind of life is that?" she asks. "You have to go out and see the beauty in things. There's a reason why when we're children our mothers were always sending us outside to play. Because that's where we thrive—out there doing something."

Annie says she has a daily routine that helps her keep her focus on what's good in her life: "I wake up every morning, stand in front of a mirror, and say, 'You are gorgeous.'"

Annie has long believed that a positive mind-set goes hand in hand with good health. "You have to put your mind to it. If you are going to wait around moping, you will find out things aren't really as great as they should be, and you'll tear yourself up in the process," she says.

Optimistic people, who credit themselves when things go well and view bad times as temporary, live longer than pessimists. According to a study conducted over a thirty-year span, pessimistic people are 19 percent less likely to reach a normal life expectancy. (Mayo Clinic 2002c)

Avoid Generational Competition

Generations see things differently because of changes in the culture, changes in events, and sometimes just because they can. Accepting different generational perspectives as a reality of life, rather than feeling a sense of rivalry with those who have different views, allows us to continue functioning in an evolving world even as we continue to value our own views.

"I HAVE EXPERIENCE. I have opinions. And I probably push too far," Lynn says in explaining why she's taking a class in grandparenting at her local community center.

Lynn told her daughter one too many times about how to dress a child or the level of table manners expected of a child. Tensions rose, and her family could seldom enjoy each other's company. "Each time, I thought I knew best," Lynn says. "I was trying to help her head off mistakes. What's the point of making a mistake if you don't have to?"

But the lessons of grandparenting class are offering a new perspective. "They say we grandparents can push for too much control," Lynn says. According to the class, she explains, "grandparents have to leave their egos at the door and not try to impose their parental perspective on their adult offspring. And we need to know that not everyone is going to see eye to eye with us. And that's not their fault."

Because of the class, "I will never again say, 'I know what to do. I raised you,'" Lynn says. "I guess it's kind of demeaning and demanding: 'Do everything my way because I've done this before.' But it's tough. I'm still having to edit myself."

Nine in ten mothers and fathers said there were significant differences in their approach to parenting compared with their own parents, and the majority said their different approaches were a source of tension. (Morman and Floyd 2002)

Drink Less

While the many health dangers of excessive alcohol consumption are well documented, the stability of relationships is also severely affected by alcohol. Long-term sustained drinking patterns affect emotional states and views of the world—leaving light drinkers happier and more confident in their relationships.

FOR STEPHEN BALDWIN, although acting is the family business, he has had to struggle against comparisons with his older and more famous brothers. While trying to make a name for himself, he has sought to portray characters on the outside looking in. "These characters have the feeling of emptiness," Stephen says. "They exude a detachment, which they use as a shield. It's a feeling they've had to create for themselves after being exposed to the worst elements of this world."

Emptiness has been all too easy to tap into for Stephen. He attributes a series of failed relationships to the problems with alcohol that he experienced in the early years of his acting career. He turned his life around a decade ago. "It feels great," he says. "I'm no longer harming myself, which means I can be there for someone else."

That someone else is Stephen's wife, Kennya. Stephen says, "The smartest thing I ever did was marry Kennya."

He adds, "There are two very important words that husbands have to learn. They are 'Yes, dear.' Marriage and fatherhood are the only true realities that I experience. I'm in this kooky business that is not rooted in reality."

Over the course of a decade, a low frequency of alcohol consumption was associated with a 57 percent greater chance of maintaining a happy long-term relationship than was moderate to heavy drinking. (Prescott and Kendler 2001)

Try Something New

We are often leery of something new—whether it's as important as a new job or a new direction in life, or as trivial as a new product in the supermarket—because we are comfortable with the old and familiar. Give yourself a chance to like new things; they won't always be what you want, but it's unlikely they won't ever be what you want.

LISA KNOWS IT'S not the typical path. "Most people, when they graduate from high school, don't ever want to come back," she says. Instead, the sixty-something mother and grandmother decided to return four decades after high school as a substitute teacher. Substitute teaching was just the thing to give her some variety in her life while still leaving her with free time.

Lisa says she likes the idea that every day is a little different, holds something new. "And I feel needed. I fill a void. It's my contribution to the world," she says.

Interacting with different generations also is energizing for her. "I really like young people," Lisa says. "They give me a fresh outlook. I like to do anything the students do. In math, which is not my strongest subject, I have great respect for their knowledge. And I learn new things in the process.

"It's exercise for my brain, and it's a joy," Lisa adds.

"I think I'm a student at heart. I have an insatiable quest for knowledge, reviewing what I studied years ago and learning new material and then teaching it," Lisa says. "It's a great way to learn.

"Sometimes when I get home from school, my friends ask, 'When are you going to stop that foolishness?' It's not foolishness. It's fun."

Those over fifty who showed a high degree of resistance to change were 26 percent less likely to feel optimistic about their futures. (Caughlin and Golish 2002)

Remember the Task, Forget the Rankings

What would be your reaction if everyone in your office was being taught a new procedure and you felt completely lost about how it worked? For most people, the answer is that they would hide their ignorance from their co-workers. For most people, more important than actually finding out what they need to know is not letting anyone know they need help. But what is your true priority? Is it to cleverly trick your colleagues into believing you know everything? Or is it to learn what you need to know to do your job well?

PAT FLYNN RUNS a small manufacturing plant in northern Virginia. Pat tries to teach his employees the difference between style and substance.

"If everybody cared about style, and not substance, nothing would get done," Pat says. "Why, we would never have had a man walk on the moon. There'd just be three guys jammed in the doorway of the space-ship, all trying to get out ahead of the others to get their picture on TV.

"The day we accept style over substance," Pat continues, "is the day we stop making products that serve any purpose, that do any good. You want style over substance, go do something that doesn't matter."

Researchers have found a fascinating change that takes place in schoolchil-dren. When they begin their studies, there is no difference between the best and worst students in terms of their willingness to ask questions when they do not understand. However, as they get older and begin to understand their relative position in the class, students, especially weaker students, become reluctant to ask questions and reveal what they do not know. (Butler 1999)

Find a Community That Fits Your Family

Where you live will be a significant influence on your life and your outlook. The community you live in can complement your journey or impede it. Seek a place to live that truly meets your needs.

EAST FARMINGTON, MINNESOTA, was designed so that a close-knit community could call it home. With University of Minnesota experts overseeing the plans, the town was literally made to bring people together. The houses sit on small lots on narrow streets, so the residents are close together physically. To encourage daily interaction, sidewalks go in every direction, the mailboxes are all clustered together, and every house has a front porch. And the backyards open onto common areas, many with shared playgrounds for kids.

Before moving to East Farmington, Claire says, she had been living in a "modern suburban isolation. You could not walk anywhere. There were no sidewalks, no crosswalks, and the roads weren't safe to cross. Children weren't allowed out of their fenced-in yards. I didn't know anyone on the block and seldom exchanged more than a nod with them." Claire moved to East Farmington to recapture a feeling she had when she was a child: "We had sidewalks; the kids ran around to their friends' houses. Everyone knew one another. There was a real community there, where people weren't isolated from each other."

Claire says East Farmington is better: "People do come together more here. I know more neighbors. It isn't perfect, but it makes you feel so much better about where you live when you feel a connection to the place and the people."

People who were highly satisfied with their neighborhood were 25 percent more likely to be highly satisfied with their family life. (Toth, Brown, and Xu 2002)

Turn Off the TV

Television is the creamy filling that distracts us from the substance of our lives. Do not let television become the default organizer of your time.

LANCE COMPARES WATCHING television to getting lost in a cave: "It may seem interesting, but you've got to get out eventually." Lance gave up television after examining whether it was worth the hours he was spending on it.

"If you add up the time in your day, especially the free time in your day, and then figure out how much goes out to television, it will make your jaw drop," Lance says. "We just don't even consider the alternatives. For most people, it would be like choosing to walk across the country instead of fly. But there's just so much freedom in your life when you gain that time."

Lance says that one of the great surprises of living without television is how much he still knows about television. "Everybody thinks they will be lost at the water cooler conversation if they don't have a television. But there is so much coverage about television—just reading the newspaper, you would know an awful lot about *Desperate Housewives* and *American Idol*."

Watching too much TV can triple our hunger for more possessions while reducing our personal contentment by about 5 percent for every hour a day we spend watching. (Wu 1998)

Honor Your Spiritual Beliefs

Discomfort in our lives comes in many shapes and sizes, but the most pressing concerns are basic matters of life and death. We desire a life well lived, and a death of grace. People with strong spiritual beliefs enjoy a strong sense of purpose in their lives and see their death as another chapter in life. Let your spiritual beliefs guide you to your ethic and to your joy.

ROBERT HAS LIVED his personal and professional life around his religion. As a Presbyterian pastor, he has mentored countless people through their lives, careers, and spiritual journeys.

Now Robert is making a major career transition of his own. With an eye toward his eventual retirement, he's sharing his church responsibilities with a young co-pastor, Brian. Robert and Brian alternate offering sermons and share the many small-group and personal counseling tasks Robert had long built into his schedule.

Brian knows that many pastors could not accept the idea of sharing their workload, their position, their church with anyone. "I have been approached in the past to be a co-pastor in other situations, and I have declined, because it really has to be a special pastor who would truly share the position. Robert has done that graciously," Brian says.

Robert sees the transition not as a threat to his ego but as a celebration of his faith. "My role is to help Brian, help the congregation adjust from me to him and to his leadership," Robert says. "It keeps the momentum going, and it keeps people's interest high. This is not about the end of my role. It's about the importance of this church in the lives of all our congregants, including my own."

Those over fifty who said they had strong spiritual beliefs were 4 percent more likely to be happy, regardless of which religion they subscribed to. (Francis, Jones, and Wilcox 2000)

Drink Grape Juice

Much as the Teflon coating keeps food from sticking to a pan, the bioflavonoid in grape juice interferes with the process by which cholesterol sticks to our arteries. Regular consumption of grape juice therefore reduces the likelihood of clogged arteries and lowers the risk for conditions including heart disease and strokes.

"BIOFLAVONOIDS, OR COMPOUNDS that act as antioxidants, fight damaging free radicals. They occur naturally in a number of foods, such as fruits and vegetables, especially apples and onions; tea, especially green tea; chocolate; nuts; grape juice and red wine," says Dr. Michael Lefevre of Pennington Biomedical Research Center

"The data suggests that bioflavonoids offer a protective effect against LDL, or the bad cholesterol, and improve endothelial function to keep the blood vessels dilated," he says.

Dr. Lefevre said it would be a good idea for people to look at their diets and determine whether they are consuming foods that contain bioflavonoids. "Food are not created equal; even foods we think of as healthy are not created equal. I try to eat a lot of green, leafy vegetables, onions, and apples. And drink things like grape juice. Grape juice is the kind of beverage that children tend to consume a lot of, and then people forget about it as they become adults. It's time to rediscover it and put a glass of grape juice in your diet every day."

In studies of people with heart disease, drinking grape juice for two weeks helped widen arteries and reduced cholesterol oxidation by more than a third. (Stanford University 2003)

APRIL 17

Get a Good Night's Sleep

When there are only so many hours in the day, and so much to do, the loser often ends up being sleep. But sleep is a crucial factor in your ability to function. It is food for your brain. You can sacrifice sleep to gain extra time, but ultimately you are sacrificing your ability to use your time with purpose and efficiency.

MATT SPENT YEARS as a fitful sleeper.

"Most people know what it's like on Monday morning when you haven't had much sleep during the weekend. Well, imagine what it might be like when you haven't had enough sleep for five years," Matt says.

Matt regularly felt sluggish: "My whole life was set in slow motion."

When he saw an ad for a research study on sleeping problems, Matt wondered if there was anything that could be done. He saw the doctors, and they asked him to sleep in the medical center for a few nights.

They videotaped and monitored his attempts at sleep and found that a breathing problem was continually waking him up, making a full night's sleep impossible. The problem can be reduced or eliminated by wearing a special mask that regulates breathing while sleeping.

For Matt, the device has meant almost a whole new life. "I work better, I'm a better husband, I enjoy everything I do more," Matt says.

Most Americans have been sleepy at their job, and two in five report making errors because of sleepiness. Inadequate sleep reduces innovative thinking by 60 percent and flexibility in decision making by 39 percent. (Harrison and Horne 1999)

Drive Safely When It's Safe

Understand that your safety when driving is not just about you but also about the other drivers. The vast majority of the more than forty-six thousand deaths due to car accidents in the United States every year are attributable to multicar crashes, not single car accidents. Avoid the mentality that you can and should drive any time you want to. Avoid driving at times that attract reckless drivers.

ROB TEACHES A defensive driving course outside of Pittsburgh. He emphasizes not just the skills of driving but the decisions of driving.

One is the choice of speed. Your speed matters, of course, but your speed relative to the other cars is crucial. "A big gap—in either direction—between your speed and the prevailing speed on a road is a recipe for disaster," Rob says. "Equally problematic are the dawdlers who cause brake lights behind to crescendo in red and the hot-shoes who try to slalom through traffic ten or fifteen miles an hour faster than anybody else. Go with the flow or get off the highway."

A second decision, Rob says, is the route: "Know the dangerous intersections, the curves that people take too fast, the streets without adequate lighting. There's no reason to put yourself in a dangerous spot when you know the roads."

And the third decision is timing: "Don't go just because you want to, go because it makes sense. We know that the presence of drunk drivers peaks later on weekend nights. And if you want to be a safe driver, you will factor in that you can't be a safe driver unless the other cars on the road are driven by safe drivers."

There is a 41 percent increase in driving fatalities throughout the United States on the night of the Super Bowl. This increase exceeds the surge in accidents on any other occasion, including New Year's Eve. (University of Toronto 2002a)

Seek a Tall Plateau, Not the Peak

People on top want to stay on top. It's not surprising. But people who reach an unsustainable achievement wind up longing for comparable outcomes long after those outcomes are no longer attainable. Set your goals not on reaching an ultimate moment that will quickly come and go, but on reaching a level of achievement that is both satisfying and sustainable.

UPSTATE NEW YORK florist Patricia Woyshner has been in the business for forty years.

She's sold flowers to tens of thousands of folks in the area, and even received one of the best assignments a florist could hope for—decorating the White House for the Christmas season. "I had to take a deep sigh. I mean, you see pictures of the place all your life, then one day you're in the Oval Office," Patricia says.

Despite the excitement, Patricia's focus remained steady on her day-to-day concerns. "My job is to run my business. I want to have something here that I can pass on to my children," she says.

She realized that although she knew everything about flowers, she was not an expert in marketing her business: "All my education was related to the floral industry. I realized that I should try to learn from other industries, because they face problems that are very similar to ours."

Patricia attended business school seminars designed to help her attract repeat business. Patricia reports that her customer base is up, and the White House even called and asked her to decorate again.

Studies of former Olympic athletes find, not surprisingly, that these athletes are very capable and highly motivated individuals. However, more than half of former Olympic athletes have trouble adapting to more traditional postathletic careers because they cannot replicate the heights of success and recognition they once enjoyed in athletics. (Sparkes 1998)

A Sense of Humor Helps

A good joke can brighten any day. In a relationship, a good sense of humor helps to make the average day more fun and to lessen the burden of the bad days. This humor must be aimed in positive directions, of course. Negative, biting jokes serve only to heighten tensions.

VIVA AND JERRY of Minneapolis have been hosting *Viva and Jerry's Country Videos* on local cable access for more than a decade. They are the Sonny and Cher of no-budget Minneapolis-area cable television. Their show is a mix of bad puns, country music, and spoofs, and it has drawn something of a cult following.

Viewers are attracted to silliness of the show. But most of all, they are lured by Viva and Jerry. Their playful banter and constant fawning over each other conveys an uncommon television image: a couple in their sixties who are clearly in love.

Though they appear gleefully happy on the show, the couple admit they aren't perfect. They argue, like all couples. "It's hard work," Viva says of marriage. "You have to learn to live with quirks."

The show is part of what keeps them going, something odd and funny—and in a strange way, meaningful—to share. Couples need that, Viva says. Which is why they spend so much time putting on a show that pays them nothing.

"It gives us something to look forward to," says Viva. "And it's given us new horizons; at our age, we're still meeting all these new people and doing things we would have never done. And all with a laugh."

When both partners in a relationship thought the other had a good sense of humor, there was 67 percent less conflict reported than in couples where neither thought the other had a good sense of humor. (De Koning and Weiss 2002)

Avoid the Second-Guess Paralysis

We make decisions, even important decisions, all the time. All of us make the best decision possible given the information we have available. But where do we go from there? "What if" questions intrigue us—it can be endlessly fascinating to imagine what might be different—but what-ifs do not serve us or help us reach the best possible outcome given the decisions we have actually made.

MIGUEL ARTETA'S FIRST taste of the moviemaking business was unpleasant and intimidating.

"Because people would do anything to get their first movie made, there was this constant, spirit-crunching pressure. Every decision you made was made to please the potential backers, and then when they decide not to give you money for the project, you go back and think about everything you changed to please them in the first place," Miguel says.

Then he came to the conclusion that the money chase was like a dog chasing his tail. "Everything was temporary until you got turned down, and then you started all over again," Miguel says. Instead, he decided that if he was really going to make his movie, it ought to be his movie. No more constant changes to attract backers: "We would only take money from people we respected, people whose opinions we felt good about."

Miguel wound up finding support for what became the critically acclaimed *Star Maps*, and later said his movie came to life only when he "stopped second-guessing" himself.

People who spend more time thinking about their "possible selves," the lives they might be leading if they had made different decisions, are 46 percent less satisfied with their career decisions than people who do not spend much time imagining what might be different. (McGregor 1999)

Eat Less, but Eat Often

When you are trying to cut back on the amount of food you eat, you'll be tempted to cut back on the number of times you eat. This strategy, however, is a recipe for failure. Eating fewer times per day reduces the efficiency of our bodies in processing food as fuel. In other words, skipping meals maximizes the caloric effect of the food we do eat.

MICHELLE HAS WON and lost battles with her weight at least four times during the past decade, dropping as much as sixty pounds—only to gain much of it back after meeting her goal and then losing the excitement of the challenge.

She's tried expensive meal plans and even visited a personal nutritionist in the past. But she wanted something with more personal involvement. Then she found a group of dieters online—who come together to share information, support, and inspiration.

She now logs in twice a day to read messages, and she participates in the weekly weigh-in. "I like to see other people dealing with similar issues and getting ideas from other people in the group," Michelle says.

Michelle has started a group discussion on the subject of skipping meals. "There is no way to make that work," she says. "Going to the gas station less often does not make your car use less gas. Eating fewer times does not make your body eat less; it just means you are even more hungry when you do eat, then you eat more, and your system is less well prepared to handle it."

A study found that people who ate five or six times a day had 5 percent lower total cholesterol and were 45 percent more likely to be able to sustain their target weight than people who ate once or twice a day. (Oxford University 2002b)

See Around Career Roadblocks

After enough time in a field, you are an expert. With this expertise, however, often comes frustration because there may not be any way for you to bring your vision into reality. Find an outlet for your expertise regardless of whether that outlet is within your workplace or in some other setting.

"ADVERTISING IS A strange line of work. It sits right at the intersection of creativity and commerce. If it's too much of one, it generally fails at being the other," Elliot says. Elliot was good at what he did, but he often felt stifled by the limits of the work. "You can take something only so far before it's too new, too different."

Elliot saw this in his own career and also saw the frustration in his colleagues. "These are some of the most creative people you could imagine, but some of them felt like they were running a race with lead weights in their pockets," he says.

Elliot realized he could not reinvent his company or the advertising industry. But he could provide a new outlet for bottled-up creativity.

Elliot opened a small gallery featuring all kinds of art and creative pieces. His first step was to invite his co-workers to bring him anything they might be secretly working on or had hidden in their garages and basements. "They responded with paintings, drawings, photos, sculptures, jewelry, handmade furniture, and things you just can't describe.

"The art is nice, and the shop is even clearing a tiny profit. But the point of it is to feel all the way alive," Elliot says.

Research on veteran teachers found that 64 percent were burdened with significant frustration at administrators' lack of interest in their views. Those who overcame their frustration typically redirected their energies toward mentoring new professionals or finding an outlet for their expertise outside their school. (Clarke 1998)

Be Engaged to Reality

The engagement period is an unrealistic point of comparison. Those who are engaged are flush with the excitement of a newly made major decision filling them with anticipation. Don't judge your own life by comparing it with unique moments that are not meant to be sustained.

VERMONT NATIVES DOUG and Gloria looked forward to their marriage, and their engagement was a dream come true for both.

Even after the divorce that followed four years later, Gloria admits they have a lot in common: "I think our qualities complement each other in many ways, but we were, and are, incompatible. There were too many points of contention."

Gloria cautions that the "pictures in your head of the perfect house with the white picket fence and the glamorous life can overwhelm all logic" when engagements occur. "Now I view marriage as more of a work in progress, and less a fantasy."

Indeed, as a freelance writer, Gloria has pondered that idea in her essays. "I'm interested in the unhealthy extremes we all too often live between," she says. "Engagement is no more a fairy tale than divorce is a prison sentence. Neither my ex-husband nor I became anarchists with green hair or anything like that after the divorce. We've lived full lives and happy lives, but not magical lives."

Psychologists find that "idealistic distortion"—the tendency to make unrealistically positive assessments of our relationship and our partner—is more than twice as great during an engagement period than it is during either the dating that precedes it or the marriage that follows it. (Bonds-Raacke et al. 2001)

You Don't Have to Get Straight A's Anymore

We all remember our first performance evaluation: report cards. We carried them home and presented them to our parents, yearning for their approval. This formative lesson of contingent approval still carries with us. But just as having to get good grades to please your parents did not instill a love of reading, having to succeed to attain the approval of someone else will not make you enjoy the process. To succeed, not just in the outcome but in the process, the effort has to be for you.

ANN ORTIZ BEGAN Ann's Turquoise with a vision, about $1,500, and plenty of patience.

Her vision was to create a unique retail store that featured clothing, jewelry, and crafts that couldn't be found anywhere else in the Topeka area—or anyplace else for that matter.

To do it right, Ann realized she had to take her time: "We've done this as a slow process, because if we tried to grow too fast, we wouldn't be able to maintain our purpose."

Ann's store is doing better than she could have imagined—and she someday might consider opening a second location when the time is right.

Ann says that opening a store "taught me that if you really enjoy and love something, it shows through your work. It's shown me what an individual can accomplish. And that what you do doesn't have to make the biggest, best business in the world to be your business, to be your dream."

More than nine out of ten people felt, when they were children, some need to demonstrate competence to earn or deserve parental love. For most, this pattern remains in adulthood as they continue to use their careers to seek approval from loved ones despite the anxiety and disappointment this pattern can produce. (Jones and Berglas 1999)

Write Down Your Thoughts

No matter how close a family may be, there must always be space for the individual. Taking the time to write down your thoughts about your life, the world—anything that's on your mind—will give you some personal space to think and feel just for yourself.

"THIS USED TO be called a diary, then a journal, now for a lot of folks it's a blog," says Professor Pat Simmons, who has studied the effects of personal writing.

"It absolutely doesn't matter whether you use a pen and paper or a computer site; the act of writing, reflecting on your day, your life, your thoughts, your feelings, has positive effects," says Professor Simmons. "People feel like they have an avenue to share the good and the bad. They feel less likely to be overwhelmed."

Professor Simmons cautions that the modern-age version of a writer's journal—the Web log, or *blog*, for short, in which personal observations are available to anyone who visits the Web site—opens your thoughts to scrutiny and feedback: "You have to decide if you want to share these thoughts. You have to decide if you want feedback. If these are private thoughts just for yourself, then keep them private. If you need a platform to share with others, use a blog.

"Some of my students have created almost a computerized version of their lives—with stories, pictures, and the kind of information that really captures where they are in their lives."

Professor Simmons herself writes every day. "I can't imagine a day without some journal time. It would be a colder, more empty day for me," she says.

Parents who make regular entries in a journal were 12 percent more likely to feel satisfied with their family life and 26 percent more likely to feel that their individual viewpoints mattered in their lives. (Brady and Sky 2003)

Fitness Is Free

T he impressive-looking exercise machines we see advertised on television make it seem like we'd better save up if we're going to start exercising. In reality, the foundation of any good exercise program needs to be no more complicated that taking a walk or a jog for free. Expensive machinery or health-club memberships are fine if you want them, but they are not required for you to have a positive effect on your health.

LINDA HAS BEEN strolling the paved paths of Oglebay Park in Wheeling, West Virginia, for twenty years, but she has more company these days.

A barrage of television and newspaper ads promoting the health benefits of walking has helped get thousands off the couch and onto trails throughout the city. The ads resulted in a 32 percent increase in the number of people who walk for at least thirty minutes, five days a week.

While Americans spent nearly $6 billion on home-exercise equipment in 2005, Linda doesn't see the need. "Walking is the nicest exercise you can do," Linda says after a brisk morning outing with her dog. "You don't have to get all kinds of equipment. You can do it with a friend. You can do it alone. You can do it as fast or as slow as you want."

Walking makes Linda feel better physically and psychologically, boosting her energy level when she is tired. "I like being outside," she adds. "And I like getting exercise without having to kill myself."

Fitness programs based on walking or jogging, and exercises that don't require equipment, such as sit-ups, have the same beneficial health effects as machine-based exercise regimens. (University of Richmond 2002)

There's No Need to Hurry

For those who marry, the age at marriage has been getting later every decade for the past one hundred years. For those who have children, the age when a person first has children has been getting later every decade for the past one hundred years. People are starting these life-altering courses later and later for many reasons, including financial pressures and a desire to obtain and maintain independence. There's no need to hurry. Relationships are not a race, and there's no prize for finishing first.

MOVIE STUDIO CHIEF Barry Diller and fashion designer Diane Von Furstenberg were, depending on the year, friends or a couple for more than twenty-five years.

"He said it first," Diane recalled. "He said, 'Wouldn't it be nice?' We always say we're going to do it, maybe Christmas, maybe my birthday, and we don't." And with that, the longtime friends decided to get married.

Off they marched on Barry's fifty-ninth birthday to city hall in New York for a civil ceremony. They had to squeeze through reporters and photographers who were tipped off to the event by friends. "There was no serious planning," Diane said, "and that's the way I like it.

"We've been together for so long, it's like we already are married. Whatever happens, though, nothing will change. We love each other. Our relationship has always been based on truth, and a trust between us. After all these years, this feels very natural."

Marrying later in life has no negative effect on satisfaction either with the relationship or with life. (Juang and Silbereisen 2001)

Volunteer to Achieve

You're busy. You don't feel there's much more you can do at work or at home. But you want to do more and feel better doing it. Take an hour this week and volunteer. Yes, give your time away. Volunteering will of course aid your community, but it also opens us up to a greater appreciation of our own lives, which enhances our motivation to do what we do as best we can.

MICHELLE RUNS AN office-supply store in a Boston suburb. She works hard to keep the business thriving, and at the end of the day, she needs a break. What does she do? She heads to the local YMCA, where she is a volunteer.

"It's challenging and exhilarating," Michelle says of her volunteer efforts to raise money to support Y programs. "I do it because I love it, I have been given a lot in this world, and I like to give a little back."

Even though she doesn't have a lot of free time, investing some of it in the Y actually makes Michelle feel better. "It reduces stress. It gives me a real boost, because when you give time to a worthy cause, you feel so good about yourself and the world in general," Michelle says.

Volunteers are 25 percent more satisfied with their jobs, have a better work ethic, and are more persistent in working toward long-term goals and rewards. (Johnson et al. 1998)

It Doesn't Matter Who Earns the Money

Your family is not a business. There are no rankings based on who earns the most. Whatever anyone does that benefits the family is good. Seeing income competitively is a dangerous distraction from what really matters to you.

SUSAN EARNS SUBSTANTIALLY more as an advertising executive than her husband does as a union organizer. When her career began to blossom in the 1990s and her income zoomed past her husband's, tensions began to surface at home. And even as she was bringing in the bulk of the income, she was also doing the bulk of the housework.

"We had quite the row over it," Susan says. Finally they worked out a truce, and her husband began doing more of the work around the house.

But her situation prompted her to wonder if women with similar marriages faced comparable conflicts. A meeting with another female executive confirmed that she wasn't alone, and Susan began discussing the matter with women in similar situations.

"I expected to find women who really ruled the household. I figured whoever has the money has the power. But women are not necessarily taking the power position even when they make the money," Susan says.

Instead, Susan found, breadwinner wives are using their financial means to create a more cooperative marriage. "When women make more money, we have the leverage to establish a true partnership," she says.

Susan thinks any man can be happy with a breadwinner-wife marriage if he believes in himself. "Men need to have a very strong self-image but not measure their self-worth by the size of their paycheck," she says.

Married couples in which the woman earns more money than the man are no more likely to experience conflict, low marital satisfaction, or divorce than couples in which the man earns more than the woman. (Rogers and DeBoer 2001)

Notice Patterns

W hat is the great common denominator of intellectual accomplishment? Great thinkers notice patterns. They see patterns no one else has thought of, patterns no one else has paid any attention to. Thinkers notice what goes with what and then consider the meaning behind those patterns.

"I DON'T CARE what you do, you have to understand how things work. Not just thinking about what you're doing, but about what you're not doing," says George Bodrock.

"Now, my business is waste. It's not glamorous, but it's important. But what we're not doing enough of is finding natural techniques to reduce waste," he says.

That's why George, of California's Ecology Farms, a commercial waste-management company, researches "vermistabilization." That's the process of using worms to transform waste into a useful product. Bodrock supervises the use of 160 million worms who eat their weight in yard waste, and in the process convert the waste into a soil nutrient.

"People are not going to give up growing lawns, gardens, and golf courses. We can take what they throw out and recycle it 100 percent," George says. He calls the worms' endless appetite for waste "the equivalent of a perpetual-motion machine.

"We can build supercomputers that can do a billion calculations a second, but when it comes to breaking down green wastes, there's no computer to do the job. But when you do it right, you not only help the earth, you'll become rich in the bargain."

Academic achievement, regardless of the subject matter, is characterized by an ability to decipher complex ideas and relationships. Experiments in language, math, and science show that the most basic building block of learning is the independent observation of patterns. (Silverman 1998)

Get Out of the Car

Driving is so much a part of most people's lives that they forget the incredible burden it can be. Few tasks require such a commitment to comprehensive concentration, as we pay attention not only to what we're doing but to what every other driver is doing, not to mention pedestrians, and anything else that might enter our path. Anything you can do to cut down your daily driving time—carpooling, relocating, planning your route—will add positive time to your day.

THE AVERAGE LOS Angeles resident spends the equivalent of three months' worth of workdays just driving to work every year. Two weeks of that time is spent sitting in stop-and-go traffic.

"Driving is one of the great eaters of time in our society," says sociologist Walter Rose. "Many of us see the freedom of driving, of going where you want when you want, but we overlook the very real costs.

"Driving time is not time that's particularly good for anything else. If you are walking or riding a bicycle, you are getting exercise. If you are taking a bus or train, you can read or work. If you are driving, you are just driving. At least, that's all you should be doing if you want to be safe."

Professor Rose says that people often make the decision to live farther from their job because they think it's a better use of their time: "They see the freedom of being right where they want to be on a Saturday morning. But they need to consider where they're going to be on Monday through Friday morning, too—which is stuck in traffic."

Every additional ten miles in a daily commute increases stress levels by 5 percent. (Lucas and Heady 2002)

It's Always a Choice

Y ou may feel like you have no option but to accept burdens on behalf of your loved ones. But every single thing you do is your choice. Draw strength from your decision to make those you care about your priority.

LIKE MANY COUPLES, Liz and James planned a magical wedding day. A huge gathering of friends and family were there to see them start their lives together. "Everything was perfect. We were living a fairy tale," James says of the time.

Ten years later, Liz and James both have demanding careers, three young children to care for, and a huge mortgage hanging over them. Liz recounts the daily rigors: "The kids are really young and very high-maintenance. I get really tired and worn out. My husband is stressed out. It's not that it's unpleasant; it's hard."

"It's easy to see how, when reality comes for you, people start to get nervous," James says. "You stop seeing all the things you did to get here, how you took steps to create this. And all you see is this great big burden."

Liz and James know that getting to their ten-year anniversary, and planning to celebrate many more anniversaries, is a decision they both make every day. "This is about dedication," James says. "You decide every day if you are dedicated to this, and if you are, there is nothing that can stop you. If you aren't, watch out, because it's not easy."

"It's a choice," Liz echoes. "You learn to see the beauty in what you choose, and realize all that you have. We are best friends, we have wonderful children, we have the life we want."

People who thought of their family life as an active choice that they made and continue to make were 77 percent more likely to feel satisfied with their family life. (Nanayakkara 2002)

It's Less What Happened Than What Happened Next

Y ou will face difficult times. Everyone does. But how things turn out for you has less to do with the events themselves than with your response. Answer the challenges that are presented to you, persevere through the traumas that may occur, and you will be made stronger for your life ahead.

DOUG HAD LOST his wife to illness only a year before. The grief was still fresh within him. When there was a knock on his door early one morning, he knew that whatever would bring someone to his home at that hour could not be good. He would learn that his brother had been killed by what the media called "the sniper," two serial killers who had been terrorizing the Washington, D.C., area in 2002.

Doug had seen the news stories, but he hadn't imagined for a moment when he heard the latest tragic report that the unnamed victim was his brother.

When his wife died, Doug figured that he could take one of two paths: he could be bitter and angry at the cruel loss, or he could accept that she was in a better place and that he would have to go on living his life. He tried to hold those thoughts as he faced the excruciating task of telling his elderly parents that their son was gone.

"It's not easy, but we still need to realize all the wonderful things we've been privileged to experience. A family is like a table, with each person a leg," Doug says. "We feel the loss, and it aches. But we're going to have to fight through this and live with a wobbly table."

The length of time personal tragedies continued to affect life satisfaction ranged from days to decades depending on the person's response to the stressors. (Hamarat et al. 2001)

Forgiveness Helps You Heal

Being able to forgive, to let go of angry thoughts and feelings, promotes the body's natural ability to return from an aroused state to a normal state. Staying at an even keel allows our bodies to function at their best. For the sake of your own health, avoid holding grudges.

DREW REMEMBERS THE feeling in the pit of his stomach every time he thought of it. A co-worker, someone he considered a close friend, had taken credit for his idea and was reaping the benefits of it at work.

"I could really work myself up every time I saw her, every time I thought about it. Just about anywhere and anytime I might start getting angry again," Drew says.

Drew noticed, however, that his anger had little effect on his friend—and a big effect on himself. "I would be steaming, and she would be sitting there, pretending nothing was wrong. Of course, for her, nothing *was* wrong," he says.

A doctor's visit confirmed Drew's suspicion that his anger was having significant effects: "My blood pressure was up, and when the doctor asked if I was under any unusual stress, I had only one explanation."

Drew decided that he could not continue to harbor anger or disappointment. While he considered the friendship irreparably harmed, he decided he could not dwell on the past or the hurt he had felt. "I started looking to the future and realized that the only way past this situation, and the only way to reducing this stress in my life, was to let it go. It's over. I learned from it, and now it's on to a better day," Drew says.

Holding a grudge raises the heart rate, blood pressure, and sweat production in more than nine in ten people. Each of these symptoms indicates an activated nervous system and increased stress hormones. (University of Maryland 2002).

There Is Plenty of Time

Whatever our dreams are, we practically hear a clock ticking. The media, our family, our friends all make us wonder when we are finally going to be "there," and why we aren't there yet. The truth of the matter is that there are no age restrictions on success. It takes as long as it takes, and when you reach it, you won't reject success because you're not the right age for it.

"THERE ARE PEOPLE on top, and then there are people who don't matter. That's how I felt," admits Nathan, who works in advertising in New York. "I suffered through every day like it was my personal humiliation.

"I didn't take pride in what I did. I practically created a fictional job for myself whenever anybody asked me what I really did.

"And in this business, there's nothing but perception. We don't make better mousetraps, we don't make anything. We sell perception, and our jobs are perception. Each day made me seem more of a failure."

Nathan sought help from a career coach, who asked him who he was really competing with, and why. He explains, "When I said I guess I was competing with everybody in the company, because I wanted to be on top, she said, 'Well, if you were on top of the company, then you'd be competing with every other company to be bigger than them.' Basically, she made me see that there was no way to win this contest, and that I could either sit back and enjoy the ride, or I would be racing to a place I could never get.

"Now I try to keep my focus on doing the best work I can, and know that I'll get where I'm going when I get there."

Age is unrelated to people's commitment to their jobs. (Tuuli and Karisalmi 1999)

Do Not Go to War with Bacteria

We have antibacterial soap, antibacterial cleaners, even antibacterial cooking surfaces. Unfortunately, the war against bacteria can actually make us weaker and the germs stronger. There is no reason to douse yourself or your home with antibacterial cleaners at every opportunity.

CLEANLINESS IS NEXT to godliness, we are taught, but is it possible to become so clean that it's not good for us? That's the question Stuart Levy, a Tufts University geneticist, has posed.

All that scrubbing and sponging with new antibacterial soaps and detergents may be weakening our immune systems, Dr. Levy says. It is killing helpful germs and spurring the growth of mutant strains of super-bacteria, he contends.

Dr. Levy longs for the days when children built strong immune systems by, in part, getting dirty. He wants us to use the cleaners our parents trusted: plain soap and water.

"Our modern obsession with protecting ourselves from every germ, every dog hair, and every fleck of dust might be backfiring. That arsenal of cleaning products in our cupboards might be our undoing. It seems that our immune systems have been so coddled by antibacterial soap and Lysol that they don't build up the musculature to fight off disease," Dr. Levy laments.

"We are fast becoming a society with an immune system so fragile that even the unpleasantness and misfortunes of daily life send us reeling," Dr. Levy warns.

Doctors have determined that much of the bacteria on the skin is protective. It is there to prevent harmful bacteria from flourishing and making you ill. If that bacteria is not there, it cannot do its job. Scrubbing with antibacterial soap removes the good bacteria with the bad. (Hackensack University Medical Center 1999)

Be Open

People in healthy relationships share what they are going through, good or bad, with their partners. Don't hold back—anything. Because in sharing your reality, you will be sharing your life, and the bond you make in the process will help you through anything.

RAOUL FELDER HAS a unique perspective on relationships. He's a happily married divorce attorney.

"I don't believe you have to be happy in what you're doing," he says. "That's a myth. I hate what I do—representing people in the most acrimonious, bitter divorces." Nevertheless, Felder spends his days representing celebrity clients as they dissolve their marriages and seek an equitable share of their marital assets. He has represented one of Johnny Carson's wives, one of Elizabeth Taylor's husbands, and Mrs. Mike Tyson.

How does Raoul Felder manage the task of being a top attorney and a dedicated family man? "In both my marriage and my career, I succeed because I am open. I am open with my wife and open with my clients. A good lawyer has to be able to write, read, and speak with total clarity, and that's very rare today," he said. "A good husband needs to do the same." A bad lawyer-client or husband-wife relationship, he says, is when "they don't know where each other is going or where they went. I'm the opposite of that."

Felder's emphasis on communication is both a commitment and a source of pleasure: "I find it easy because I appreciate the glory of the English language."

In studies of marriages of various lengths, couples with a high degree of intimacy between the spouses—that is, couples who shared their innermost thoughts—were 62 percent more likely to describe their marriage as happy. (Pallen 2001)

Home Means More Than Work to Your Health

Conventional wisdom has it that work stress can be the main hurdle to living a healthy life. For most people, however, home life is a far more significant factor in overall health than work life. The positive effects of a good home life are more powerful than the negative effects of a bad work life.

BRIAN AND CLARE are in a unique position to compare the stress of home life to the stress of work life. For the first ten years after Brian graduated from law school, he was on the fast track. He worked six days a week and never even thought of taking a vacation. He found his match in Clare, whose office was down the hall and who matched him hour for hour in dedication to her job.

In their few spare hours a week away from work, Brian and Clare began dating. Two years later they were married.

When Clare got pregnant, Brian started having thoughts about dedicating himself to his family life full-time. "Clare was clear that she didn't feel like she was finished with what she was doing. She wanted to cut back, but not cut out," Brian says. So, Clare says, Brian "changed a lot of diapers and learned more lullabies than he ever imagined existed."

Even though their days are completely different, their nights and weekends are entirely the same. And their commitment to each other and the baby is complete. And how has the arrangement affected their health? "We both recently had checkups, and we both came through with flying colors," Clare adds.

Researchers who studied the effects of work and marriage on health found that the strain of a person's job was unrelated to long-term blood pressure. Those with strong marriages, though, showed an 8 percent improvement over time. Those with struggling marriages, conversely, deteriorated by 6 percent. (University of Toronto 2002b)

Balance Depends on Which Way You Lean

We all know that we should strive to balance our lives. We need to do things in moderation. But what that means you should do to improve your life differs depending on which direction you lean. Long workdays and career priorities cry out for a different response than does a total focus on family and relationships. Create the balance that levels your life.

HE WRITES, DIRECTS, helps run a theater company he's a founding member of, and, in his spare time, starred as Ross in the television hit *Friends*. But David Schwimmer also recognizes the limits of his work. "I find it sad that everyone wants their fifteen minutes of fame and we are so consumed by it. It has never been comfortable to me," David says.

One thing he had in common with his character, Ross, he says, was depth: "Not everything is frivolous to Ross. There's a seriousness about him in terms of how he thinks about relationships, the family."

Nonetheless, David says there is a void in his life where a relationship and family belong: "I'm a workaholic, and that has gotten in the way. I have not been able to find a healthy balance between my work life and my personal life. It's a flaw in my personal character, and I can't seem to find the balance yet." He hopes that balance may come now that *Friends* has finished its course. "My time will come, and my life will change," David says.

Studies find that the balance between work life and personal life is consistently different for men and women. Most women express more satisfaction with their family as they work more hours outside of the home. Most men express less satisfaction with their family life as they work more hours outside of the home. (Marks et al. 2001)

Buy Fun, Not Stuff

If you had some money and could buy either an item or an experience, which would you buy? Most people think the item would have greater lasting value because you could use it again and again, while the experience would be something that comes and goes. But experiences such as trips, events, and classes provide shared memories that can last a lifetime and have far greater impact over time than items you can purchase.

ANN IS A retail consultant who studies what people spend their money on. Increasingly she sees people turning from ordinary gifts to intangible, experiential gifts.

"I think the most important part is the potential to make a memory," she says. "There are countless experience gifts that will literally never be forgotten. It doesn't have to be sending someone to an exotic location. You could get them a cooking lesson where they have fun, learn some things, and think of you every time they make that dish. You could get someone a balloon ride or a visit to the spa. The only common denominator is that it is something you do."

Ironically, Ann sees the rise of gifts you experience tied in part to the wide array of physical gifts available. "Try to buy an electronic gift for someone and you could spend the rest of your life studying the options, only to find out you bought something incompatible with what the person already has. Or what you bought was the latest thing for a week, but then it's outdated. It's just overwhelming, and whatever you buy could easily get lost in the clutter of the recipient's life," Ann says.

Psychologists have found that people are 44 percent more likely to think fondly of trips and other experiences they bought than of similarly priced items. (Van Boven 2005)

Happy Looks for Happy

We see far too many things every time we step outside the door to focus on all of them. Understand that you can get all the supporting evidence you want regardless of whether you start today determined to think the worst of the world or determined to think the best.

THE BREEZE COMES in softly as the sun sets. Chris looks out, and as far as the eye can see he views the calm blue ocean. In the distance, he surveys the ships passing miles out from the coast. Chris works at a Florida lighthouse. Chris came to the lighthouse after serving more than two decades as a New York City firefighter.

He wasn't on duty on September 11, but he raced into the city to try to serve. Reaching the Twin Towers after they had collapsed, he found a devastated area that looked like a war zone. The ash and smoke were overwhelming.

It was spooky, Chris says, because there were fire trucks everywhere, but no firemen. Only later did he realize the nature of the devastation suffered by the fire department, including the loss of one of his closest friends.

He mourned, feeling survivor's guilt and slipping deeper into gloom. Everywhere in the city, including his home, were reminders of that day. He left the department—not to forget, but to find another way.

Then Chris and his family decided that a move to Florida was the right thing to do. Now he takes solace in the rhythms of a new work routine, meeting new neighbors, and doing some of the unique things you can do in Florida, like going kayaking in January.

Researchers who studied people's level of interest in and attention to strangers found that people who were sad spent 35 percent more time focusing on strangers who looked unhappy. (Gotlib et al. 2004)

Ask Whether a Medicine Is Right for You

The effectiveness of all kinds of medical treatments are based on over-all averages. That is, a good treatment is one that has been effective for the average person in the past. Your particular situation may not fit that average, however. Whether you are choosing an over-the-counter medicine or receiving a prescription from your doctor, ask whether the medicine is meant for someone in your precise situation.

"DESPITE MOUNTING EVIDENCE showing that men and women respond differently to the same drug, most physicians and their patients are still not aware that sex matters when prescribing medications. In this case, we know there's a difference, and too many in the health-care field pretend that there's not," says Sherry Marts, scientific director of the Society for Women's Health Research.

Why the lack of awareness? One of the reasons is that the Food and Drug Administration and the pharmaceutical industry, groups responsible for drug labeling, only recently began to analyze safety data by gender. In fact, the reporting of gender-based data analysis in medical journals, while increasing, is still not routine practice, according to Dr. Marts. This shortcoming of the system keeps gender-specific risks as well as benefits buried beneath heaps of data.

So what can you do to protect yourself from potentially harmful drugs? Dr. Marts says, "We all must demand that physicians and pharmacists fully inform us about the pharmaceuticals prescribed and their applicability to our precise condition."

Forty percent of medicines tested had significantly different effects on women than they did on men. (Stanford University 2002b)

Beware of Fairy Tales

Our first conceptions of relationships, love, marriage, and life happily ever after are powerfully influenced by classic stories we read and films we saw. See the magic of everyday life, of sharing and caring about someone, but don't riddle yourself with expectations of a fairy tale where the story is strictly about the search for love and the rest of life is just supposed to figure itself out.

"IT'S A WAR against normal people, normal lives, fulfillment, and just about everything else that's good and reasonable," says media critic Sharon Tarver.

Her target—media depictions of relationships.

"We have one basic model out there," says Sharon. "The *Sleepless in Seattle* model, or just about any Meg Ryan movie for that matter, where the perfect person is out there, just waiting to meet you, if only you could find them. Or even worse, *Kate and Leopold,* where her character needs to travel back in time to the 1800s to find someone worthy. The message here is that solid, upstanding citizens all around you need not apply. There's somebody perfect out there.

"And look at the poll results. Ninety-four percent of people in their twenties set their sights on finding their ideal soul mate to marry. Their ideal soul mate! It's chilling, really. The message is 'Don't get married, don't get in a committed relationship—because perfection awaits.'"

Sharon implores people to understand that "Cinderella, Prince Charming, Meg Ryan—these are not real people. Don't get trapped by the sales pitch for them."

Elements of fairy tales such as Cinderella were present in 78 percent of people's beliefs about romantic love. Those people were more likely to have experienced disillusionment, devastation, and angst in their relationships than were those who gave less credence to fairy tales. (Lockhart 2000)

Lessons Can't Threaten

Why would anyone be against learning something that might make their job easier? Often it is because they fear that anything that might make their job easier might one day be able to do their job. Teaching is like asking someone to go on a trip. No one is going to take you up on an invitation to travel on a trip from which they would never return. When you try to teach anyone something new, you have to make it clear from the outset that the destination is someplace we'd all like to go.

"WHAT DO I need that for?" Jack protested when his granddaughter asked why he didn't use a computer. Jack had been a farmer all his life and had gotten along fine for fifty years without using a computer.

His granddaughter gave him twenty examples of things he could do with a computer—keep track of his expenses, plan his growing schedule—and each time Jack replied that he been doing those things without a computer.

"What about the weather?" his granddaughter asked. "What about reports you could get in an instant?"

Finally Jack relented, and a seventy-year-old farmer who had never so much as set his VCR was using a computer to track every aspect of his farm. Jack admits that old habits die hard: "I get stubborn, like anybody else. I don't need every newfangled thing to do this job, but every now and then a piece of equipment does help."

Feelings of self-threat are the single biggest obstacle to gaining the willing participation of workers in new training programs. Moreover, feelings of self-threat tend to spread among co-workers as they share their concerns. (Wiesenfeld, Raghuram, and Raghu 1999)

Stay in Control

Your life is the consequence of your decisions. Regardless of your life situation, you have to see that your decisions matter. While accountability and responsibility are heavy burdens, the most important thing that accompanies a belief in consequences is freedom.

RUDY HAS SPENT a four-decade career mentoring high school students as a teacher, counselor, and coach.

"The number one thing I tell kids—and it doesn't matter what context we're talking about—is that their decisions matter," Rudy says. "You don't want to study—that decision matters. You go out when you should be home—that decision matters. You goof off during practice instead of working hard—that decision matters.

"You have to be able to see cause and effect. Otherwise, even if you want the right effect, you won't know how to cause it."

Rudy has seen former students improve in school, head off to college, and succeed in careers. He says there is no better tribute to his personal belief that decisions matter than when he gets a note or a visit from a former student telling him they wouldn't be where they are today without him.

Feeling that their lives were beyond their control reduced the likelihood of life satisfaction by 40 percent and contributed to feelings of despondency in eight out of ten people surveyed. (Nair 2000)

Use the Stairs

Improving your health can be as simple as changing a few habits. For one, take the stairs every day instead of the escalator or elevator. Tiny acts like this in the course of a day can have a huge effect when we engage in them over the long term.

NEARLY SIX IN ten people experience no daily exercise.

"In many places, we've lost the ability to walk somewhere," laments Professor Harold Burton, who teaches exercise science at the State University of New York at Buffalo. "Because there are no sidewalks, or you would have to cross eight lanes of traffic, walking can be impossible. Meanwhile, with remote controls and computers, we can have just about anything we want without even getting out of our chair."

Physical inactivity is at such a strong point for him that he suggests doing any sort of extra physical activity throughout the day. "Insignificant as it may sound, when shopping, park at the far end of the lot instead of cruising around for the closest space. Get rid of the remote control so that changing the channel means getting off the couch. Take a few flights of stairs instead of making the whole trip in the elevator," Professor Burton suggests.

"If you haven't been doing any physical activity, anything you do will help you a lot," he says. "Is it as good as working out for thirty minutes, three days a week? No. But it's much better than no exertion at all."

Researchers have found that spending ten minutes on the stairs each day can result in losing ten pounds of weight over the course of a year. The Centers for Disease Control and Prevention encourages employers to make stairways more attractive and interesting by adding artwork to the stairways, a move that they found can increase stair usage 14 percent. (Centers for Disease Control and Prevention 2000)

The Future Matters More Than the Past

When a relationship has a successful history, some may imagine that the work has already been accomplished. But the task of a successful relationship never ends, because the point of a relationship is to build toward the future, not the past.

THERE HAVE BEEN seventy Valentine's Days since Meyer and Nellie met. And sixty-eight years since they married. But that didn't stop Meyer from navigating the streets outside their New York City retirement center to buy his wife a box of chocolates on February 14.

"We've never stopped caring for each other," Nellie explains with pride. "He's always been my guardian."

A formal dinner was held recently at their retirement center to honor Meyer and Nellie for being the longest-married couple in New York City.

In fact, their relationship began when Herbert Hoover was president and the country was in the throes of the Great Depression. "We weren't thinking of depressions then," Nellie says. "We had other things in mind."

Despite their rich past together, Nellie thinks their relationship has prospered in the here and now. "It's as simple as this," Nellie says. "We love each other!"

After sitting in the retirement home's reception room during the afternoon, posing for photographers on hand to mark the occasion, the couple decided to return to their apartment to rest for their big night. "Come on kiddo," said Meyer, playfully, before helping her up; "let's go upstairs."

Satisfaction in a relationship is eight times more reliant on recent feelings and the ability to perceive improvements than it is based on the history of the relationship. (Karney and Frye 2002)

Listen to Your Favorite Music

A song is so much more than sound to us. It is a feeling, a memory, a new world, or a trip back to an old world. Keep music in your life wherever you go.

SOME HAD NEVER played before in their lives. Others have been tinkering around with an instrument for decades.

They have two things in common: they all love music, and they all are over fifty.

Members of the New Horizons Band, a national network of fifty-and-over amateur musicians, have organized more than one hundred chapters across the country.

"It's like a runner's high," says Peter, a retired doctor and trumpet player. "Endorphins get released. You don't want to go to bed after we play."

While many band members have to deal with some physical limitations, they all persevere. "With peripheral vision on the decline, it makes it harder for the musicians to watch the conductor," says Bob, who serves as a conductor for three Atlanta-area New Horizons bands. With diplomacy, Bob says that such conditions make for "interesting times. Every performance is different." But as one band member says of Bob, "He has a knack for telling you you're playing very badly without making you feel bad."

Senior players also enjoy advantages. Bob says, "They really want to play, and they have a lifetime of music in their heads. That's a fantastic resource to draw from."

"It's a great escape," Peter says. "When you're here you can forget your other worries and troubles and get lost in the music."

In various studies, nearly all participants showed improved mood and feelings of satisfaction when their favorite music was played for them. (Burack, Jefferson, and Libow 2002)

Separate Hype from Substance

When we go shopping for a car, we have our defenses ready when the used-car salesperson greets us. We know to separate out the fluff and be wary of claims made about the perfect condition of the car and its kindly former owner, who rarely drove it. But in the field of medicine, the importance of the topic actually leaves us more vulnerable to foolhardy claims. We need to bring our skepticism with us, however, even when we desperately want easy answers to our important health concerns.

"PATIENTS WITH CANCER and other life-threatening conditions often turn to complementary or alternative medicine for a variety of reasons, and a major source of their information is the Internet," says Dr. Scott Matthews of the University of California, San Diego. However, he cautions, "there is a staggering amount of medical misinformation on the Internet."

Dr. Matthews and his colleagues reviewed 194 Internet sites with information on alternative medicine treatments. In their review of the Internet sites, the researchers looked at whether the treatments were for sale online, whether the sites provided "patient testimonials," whether the treatment was touted as a "cancer cure," and whether the treatment claimed to have "no side effects."

A "yes" answer to any of the questions raised a red flag for the researchers, suggesting that the Internet site's scientific accuracy was questionable. The researchers found that up to 90 percent of the sites raised at least one red flag.

Patients who have read of Dr. Matthews's study have thanked him, he says, for "helping them weed out some of the danger and the make-believe in health information."

More than 60 percent of Internet users visit Web sites for health advice, and more than 90 percent believe that the advice they find there is reliable. (Tufts University 2003)

It Starts and Ends with You

All commerce began with people offering goods and services by themselves. In the beginning, everyone in business was in business for themselves. Although we now live in a world with massive, international corporations that can grow bigger than a country, many yearn for the freedom and personal responsibility of running their own operation. But even if you never step out on your own, you will be making highly significant decisions about where you want to be and what you want to do. Accept personal responsibility for these decisions, and prepare yourself for the potential opportunities of the future.

"IF YOU HAVE the ability, believe in yourself, and can conceive it, then you have to have the determination to do it," says Dr. Bernard Harris, a veteran of multiple space-shuttle flights and over 4 million miles of space travel.

Harris grew up in Gallup, an isolated village in New Mexico. But his dreams were limitless when he saw the Apollo missions on television.

Before becoming an astronaut, Dr. Harris went to medical school and then joined the air force as a flight surgeon.

"Nobody from Gallup has an easy path paved to success. You have to make your own way. And I never let anyone tell me I couldn't do something," says Dr. Harris.

He frequently shares stories of his life with schoolchildren. He tells them there is only one way he could get the chance to fly in space: "Your attitude determines your altitude."

The ability to accept personal responsibility for work outcomes and to thrive under individual scrutiny improves your chances by 65 percent of successfully making the transition from a traditional job in a large company to succeeding in a job at a small firm or as an independent consultant. (Peiperl and Baruch 1997)

See the Big Picture

We often let one frustration block out our vision of everything else. When you feel defeated by a problem, step back from the situation and look at your life with a longer-range perspective.

"IF YOU LOOK closely enough, everything can be seen as an obstacle," says Kelly, who works as a job counselor and is raising two children. "It's easy to get caught up in every problem you have—to race from one thing to the next and never really see where you are going."

Kelly says that habit undermines our ability to persevere: "It becomes so much easier to think 'It's impossible,' 'It's not worth my time,' 'Let someone else do it' when you are not in touch with your larger purpose."

Both as a parent and a counselor, Kelly tries to encourage an attitude of feeling capable, motivated, and responsible. And to do that, she emphasizes the importance of thinking big.

"Everybody knows how to make decisions that instantly please them," Kelly says. "What's important is to learn to think beyond that. When you learn to balance your natural tendency to live for today with a long-term vision, you can start really planning for what you want—and valuing the things that will pay off in the long term, whether they be family, school, work, or anything you are dedicated to."

Within families, Kelly recommends that adults share their experiences, their life history: "Nothing makes the reality of long-term causes and effects real like a person who has lived them. Tell the stories of how you persisted in the face of temporary frustrations, and you are sharing the big picture and making it easier for others to appreciate what they need beyond today."

Satisfaction with life is nine times more strongly affected by a feeling of general life quality than by specific events or challenges in life. (Symmonds-Mueth 2000)

Make Your Work a Calling

I f you see your work as only a job, then it's dragging you away from what you really want to be doing. If you see it as a calling, then it is no longer a toiling sacrifice. Instead, it becomes an expression of you, a part of you.

VICTOR IS A motorman for the Chicago Transit Authority. Five days a week he's running an elevated train on the Red Line. Victor stands out in the minds of the people who ride his train because of a notable and unusual trait: he loves his job.

"Thank you for riding with me this evening on Electric Avenue. Don't lean against the doors, I don't want to lose you," he tells passengers over the intercom as the train departs.

As the train makes its way north, Victor points out notable sights, including which connecting buses are waiting in the street below.

People compliment him all the time, telling him he's the best motorman in Chicago.

Victor admits, "Our equipment may be junky, but for a couple bucks, I want to give a Lincoln Town Car ride."

Why does Victor have such a positive approach to his job? "My father is a retired motorman, and one day he took me to work with him and I was so impressed looking out that window," he says, speaking of seeing the city skyline. "Ever since I was five years old, I knew I wanted to run the trains."

People who felt their work was a reflection of themselves were 39 percent more likely to say they were satisfied with their lives. (Freed 2004)

Stretch

Do your body a favor and stretch every day. It's not exciting. It seems like the kind of thing you would do before running a race. But it is important on a daily basis to give your body a stretch to help improve your circulation and prevent injuries.

SUE SAYS SHE learned the importance of stretching at an early age: "My father was a competitive gymnast. Of course, stretching was an absolute necessity for him before he began to subject his body to those kinds of strains.

"Growing up, we had a miniature gym at home in the basement with rings, weights—the whole thing. He taught us from about as far back as I can remember the importance of stretching in a serious manner before you begin to exercise."

Sixty years later, stretching is still a part of Sue's daily routine. "First thing in the morning before breakfast I do thirty minutes of stretching in my bedroom. I'm exhilarated afterward. You're aware of your body opening up, of being alive," Sue says.

Sue thinks too few people appreciate the value of stretching. "It seems so passive, people doubt it does any good. But the parts of you that need stretching are not on the surface. The good it does is very real, even if you can't see it. A good stretching routine will not only help you heal if you get injured, it will help you avoid injury in the first place," she says.

Studies of people over fifty found that those who stretched frequently were 11 percent more likely to say they felt healthy. (McAuley et al. 2000)

You Need to Know More Than Just How Talented You Are

All of us will suffer blows to our self-esteem when we fail. Regardless of how strong our beliefs are, negative outcomes will shake us. That is why you must realize not just how capable you are, but who you are. Faith in your integrity and your humanity will survive any attack based on a failure or even a series of failures. It will survive these events and give you something to start from as you rebuild your self-esteem.

PETER SHANE IS the dean of the University of Pittsburgh Law School.

He tells his graduates that after learning the law, and even achieving confidence in themselves, their education is not complete: "You will need more. You will need courage, especially if you are going to be a leader in the settings where you live, work, and worship. If you advocate change, you will have to understand that there is no change so small that it threatens no one."

The dean tells students that the world is filled with temptations to "cut corners" and to "take the path of least resistance." To overcome those temptations, he tells them, they must see their actions as examples for others: "There is no greater measure of the example you provide as a leader, as a lawyer, as a citizen, or as a parent than the decency with which you treat other human beings. This is true whether you're dealing with a friend or foe, colleague or opponent, superior or subordinate."

If they follow this path, Dean Shane tells them, they will have "the luxury of looking back on a life well-lived."

Self-esteem, by itself, does not predict success. In fact, those with particularly high self-esteem are 26 percent more vulnerable to failures and setbacks because of the devastating consequence negative outcomes can have on their self-image. (Coover and Murphy 2000)

Ask Where Your Water Comes From

Water is the healthiest drink. It contains no calories and is necessary for our bodies to function. The importance of water, unfortunately, has led to great hype and endless sales pitches. Water from the tap and pricey bottled water from a store have the same health benefits and sometimes are exactly the same thing.

THE MOST POPULAR water in California supermarkets failed to meet state water-quality standards in one-third of the samples tested and failed to meet advertised claims of purity in 100 percent of the samples tested. The Environmental Law Foundation analyzed the water and issued a report stating, "Despite state regulations meant to ensure that all vended water meets stringent health standards, buying water is like playing a slot machine: You can't be sure what will come out."

"It's very clear from our findings that the inflated prices that consumers in California pay for water is a rip-off," says Bill Walker, a coauthor of the report. "You can't just go around making claims for your product you can't meet. They should either improve their process, or they should have to stop making that marketing claim.

"The consumer pays money to get better water than tap water, and they are not getting better water than tap water," he says. "If you are buying water, research it. Find out where it comes from and what they do to it before it gets to you. Otherwise, you are paying for nothing."

Bottled water is selling at a record pace as more than half of Americans are trying to drink more water because of the health benefits associated with water. Researchers discovered, however, that 40 percent of the bottled water sold in the United States is tap water. (Natural Resources Defense Council 2002)

You Don't Have to See Eye to Eye on Everything

R elationship success does not depend on both partners seeing things the same way. Respect for the other person's perspective is far more important than constant agreement with it.

WHEN PSYCHOLOGISTS ASKED longtime married couples what's missing from wedding vows, many of the responses had something to do with understanding and respecting differences.

"I vow to understand and accept the fact that it is OK to agree to disagree," suggested Mary, a study participant. "It took me a long time to realize, 'Oh we don't have to agree on everything.'"

It really bothered Mary when she couldn't make her husband completely agree on something that mattered to her. Now, after two decades of marriage, she says, "It saves time and creates a better relationship when neither one of us has to try and change the other person.

"I think about it this way: Who is exactly like you? Who agrees with absolutely everything you think? You. Just you. That's it. But you are not married to yourself, you are married to another person. And for every idea of yours that you want appreciated, respected, or at least tolerated, there are ideas of your spouse you will have to put up with."

Couples who shared many opinions were no more likely to positively rate their communication habits or relationship overall than were people who had fewer opinions in common. (Dufore 2000)

Have a Tomato Any Way You Like

While most fruits and vegetables have dramatically different nutritional value depending on the form in which we eat them (cooked versus processed versus raw), the tomato retains its health effects in any form. Including some form of tomato product in your diet at least five times a week significantly reduces the risk of many major diseases.

"'AN APPLE A day keeps the doctor away,' the old saying goes. But it's probably time to acknowledge a tomato a day is even better," says Dr. Roger Mason. "New research is continually expanding our understanding of the positive health effects of tomatoes."

Dr. Mason says that lycopene, an organic component that turns the tomato red, is the key ingredient that links tomato consumption to the reduction of certain cancers and heart disease. Dr. Mason explains, "Lycopene is an antioxidant—a substance that protects the body from cell and tissue damage.

"Better yet, it's not just a raw tomato that scores high on the health charts. Processed tomato sauces, used in pizza and on spaghetti, may be even better at warding off some diseases than the tomato slices in your salad. This means that the tomato in the forms people already like to eat the most is a tremendous health tool."

In fact, cooked tomatoes contain as much as two and a half times as much lycopene. "Everybody thinks if you process food, you lower the nutritional value. But as it turns out, that is not always the case," Dr. Mason says.

Five servings of tomatoes a week—in any form, canned, raw, cooked, in soups, sauce, ketchup, or juice—provide enough lycopene to cut the risk of cancer and heart disease in half and to improve the health of lungs, eyes, and the skin. (Cornell University 2002a)

Success Is Formula, Not Fantasy

Watch a movie or a TV show and see what makes people successful and happy. It's usually some almost magical quality or event.

In real life, the main difference between people who achieve and people who do not isn't as exciting or mysterious, but it is as important. It is simply conscientiousness. People who approach things with order, common sense, consistency, and persistence will ultimately succeed.

IN THE EARLY 1950s, Lillian Vernon spent $500 on her first advertisement. She offered monogrammed belts and handbags, and when she was finished filling the first round of orders, she had made a $32,000 profit.

From her first successful ad to fifty years later, Lillian Vernon has been selling household items and gifts, and steadily expanding her sales. Her company now generates more than $250 million in sales every year and is one of the fifty largest companies owned by a woman in the United States.

Lillian met with her share of skeptics: "There were naysayers along the way, but I couldn't be defeated. Because all it really takes is common sense, intelligence, and hard work." Which for the seventy-one-year-old businesswoman still means a six-day work week.

Employee conscientiousness was five times more likely to predict supervisor satisfaction than was employee intelligence. (Fallon et al. 2000)

Accentuate the Positive in All Aspects of Your Life

Logically, our feelings toward our relationship, our job, our family, and our friends should be independent things. Logic does not always rule our feelings, though. Dwelling on the negative side of part of your life will encourage you to dwell on the negative side of your relationship. Emphasizing the positive aspects of your life will encourage you to see positives in your relationship.

HIS NAME IS Jason. He's twenty-six. He's good-looking. He's a software programmer with a master's degree. He loves music and movies, and he's very well read. He's churchgoing, family oriented, thoughtful.

And he hasn't been out on a date in quite some time. He's pretty sure it has something to do with the wheelchair he's in.

Many disabled people say their desire for romance and family is no different from anyone else's, yet their opportunities can be limited.

"It's hard to get people to think of you in a dating light," Jason says. "There is a tendency in our society to put people in boxes, and if you have a disability, the disability becomes the defining attribute. I'm a human being who happens to have some coordination issues from an injury. To me, this is just part of being Jason."

A friend of Jason's who also has a disability gave him this advice: live your life, feel good about who you are, but don't be too optimistic about dating.

"I understood, but that's a terribly negative view," says Jason. "I envision myself being married and having a family."

When asked first to discuss negative aspects of their lives, people were 28 percent more likely to say something negative about their relationship than they were when asked first about positive aspects of their lives. (Caughlin and Huston 2002)

Efficiency in Everything

E very organization suffers some waste. Nothing kills our initiative as quickly as the feeling that what we do doesn't matter. An organization that wastes important resources, wastes the efforts of its workers, is an organization that will waste your motivation.

"WELCOME TO THE future of farming," says Rhode Island's Michael Lydon as he surveys his greenhouse.

Inside the quarter-acre facility, Michael grows as many tomatoes as the typical farm would produce on twenty times as much land. Other farmers "are very dependent on weather conditions," Michael says. "They are very dependent on water supply. They battle insects, they battle disease. They have to waste a lot of their time and money fixing problems they can't control. I have none of these problems."

Michael was an engineer before he began farming. And he looked at farming from an engineer's perspective, trying to root out waste and increase production. "Greenhouse farming is more about quality control, so my skills adapted very well to this business," Michael says.

While the greenhouse is more productive than traditional farms during the growing season, Michael also benefits from a much longer season because his crops are protected from nighttime chills. For much of the year, his are the only local tomatoes on the produce-store shelves. And unlike tomatoes that are picked before they ripen so that they don't spoil on the trip across the country, Michael's tomatoes are picked when they ripen and taken straight to the markets.

Michael predicts that the future of farming will be inside a greenhouse: "If you want to stay in farming, and consistently produce a product, your farming has to be done in a greenhouse."

Corporate inefficiency reduces job satisfaction by 21 percent and increases employees' desire to find new employment. (Melnarik 1999)

Self-Protection Prevents Self-Reflection

If we overstate our own role in a success, we will be ill prepared to repeat the things that actually produced the success. Similarly, if we ignore our own role in an unsuccessful effort, we will fail to think about and learn from our own mistakes.

MANY PEOPLE CONSIDER Paul Baran the "father of the Internet."

Paul was an engineer for the Rand Corporation in the 1960s, and he played a major role in conceiving of the packet-switching process that was central to the development of the Internet.

Paul, who immigrated to the United States from Poland when he was a small child, tried to sell his conception of the Internet to major communication companies. They were uniformly uninterested. He recalls executives dismissing him immediately: "Imagine them listening to this young guy and saying, 'Listen, now, squirt ...'"

Paul did not give up on himself or his idea and instead realized that what he needed was not a different product or sales pitch, but a different audience.

He eventually found that when he presented his ideas to the U.S. military, where the potential for what he was offering was appreciated.

Paul is quick to share the credit for his efforts: "The Internet represents the work of thousands of people—each of us had a little piece." And thirty years after he helped get the Internet off the ground, he's still dreaming up big ideas that turn into very profitable operations: "I start these companies, then I find somebody smarter than myself to run them, and I get the hell out of the way."

When people are asked to attribute successes and failures, to explain how things happened, they are seven times as likely to focus on the significance of their efforts when describing a success as they are when describing a failure. (Moeller and Koeller 2000)

Ambivalence Is a Negative

When we are not sure, we often put off making a decision. This happens in all phases of life, including our relationships. The difference is that ambivalence about which shoes to buy doesn't affect the health of the shoes. Ambivalence about a relationship, conversely, eats away at the relationship because it represents the absence of definite positive feelings. And that absence of a positive is a negative.

DOROTHY AND RICHARD were married in 1938. They were barely out of high school and facing the continuing hard times of the Great Depression in southern Ohio.

"All our friends didn't think it would last," Dorothy says. "We were so young, it surprised us all. But I guess I was just young enough and dumb enough that I didn't have any doubts."

If the couple might have been foolhardy about anything, it was the economic realities of the time. "When we were married the first few years, things were tough, but we had each other," she says.

It was far from easy. Richard recalls, "When we got married, we didn't have anything. With our budget at the end of payday, we had fifty cents left over to spend. We went to the movies once or twice, but that was a luxury.

"But struggle can bring you closer together. We just loved each other enough and stayed together. We went through such hard times. But we never doubted each other, we never asked why we didn't have something. We had each other, and there was nothing greater than that."

One of the best predictors of future divorce among recently married couples is the expression of ambivalent feelings. Couples where one or both partners mentioned any feelings of ambivalence were three times as likely to divorce within four years. (Huston et al. 2001)

Let Your Stress Out

To appear strong, we often try to hide our struggles. But keeping our problems locked within us serves only to isolate us from people who care about us and who want to help us. The less willing you are to share your problems with loved ones and friends, the more those problems will come to overwhelm you. And the greater effect those problems will have on your life and your health.

PETE IS AN employment counselor who helps people who have lost their jobs through downsizing. Over time, Pete and his industry in general have expanded their focus from job skills and placement services to the status of the job seekers themselves. "We recognized the incredible stress this situation can create," Pete says. "And we really have to deal with the person and their feelings, or all the training in the world isn't going to see them through to their next job.

"Jobseekers and their partners tend to fall into certain emotional patterns after the job loss. Jobseekers often feel embarrassed and defensive about being unemployed and may act guarded and withdrawn. They might not want to talk about the search for fear of worrying their partner."

Pete says, "Communication is the key to making it through tough times. Open, well-organized, and active families generally do best in weathering a job loss because they can be honest and free about what they are going through and share both the difficulty and the recovery from it. Be up-front with friends and relatives. It's something that can make you or break you, and there's no advantage to going it alone."

Men who cope with stress by talking about their problems and frustrations and confiding in colleagues and friends rather than bottling things up have higher sperm counts than those who do not. (University of Missouri 2002)

Tomorrow Will Be a Better Day
(but How Exactly?)

What do you want? Most of us have plans and ideas. But the breakdown between turning our ideas and our plans into reality happens because little of what we think about progresses beyond concepts and opinions. Of course, we can never measure ourselves against concepts and opinions, because they are too abstract to define. Thus, we can't say whether we're making progress or what we need to change. Define your goals and your plans to attain them.

NANCY IS A consultant who works with small businesses.

Nancy's job is to help the owners of these business develop a map for their future. She meets with her clients once a month to talk about where they are and where they are going. "Too many small-business owners spend time dealing with one crisis after another, rather than managing their business well. There's no time for thought, no time for progress—just time to do what has to be done today.

"The toughest hurdle," Nancy says, "is just getting started in setting concrete goals so that the business can serve the long-term needs of the owner, rather than the owner spending all his time serving the short-term needs of the business."

People who construct their goals in concrete terms are 50 percent more likely to feel confident they will attain their goals and 32 percent more likely to feel in control of their lives. (Howatt 1999)

There's No Better Time to Be Sick

Many folks imagine that if they are feeling ill on the weekend, they should tough it out until Monday, when the real doctors will be at work. Although the size of a medical staff on-duty at any time varies with the typical workload of the time period, the quality of medical care does not depend on the day and time treatment begins.

"I'VE HAD PATIENTS say to me that the pain started in the middle of the night, but they didn't think about getting help until the next morning," Dr. Terry Brown says. "I wish they would understand this isn't like waiting until Monday to call the plumber so you don't have to pay overtime rates. We're here all the time, and the sooner you call us, the sooner we can help.

"People really need to separate out emergency services from their view of everything else," Dr. Brown says. "Police, the fire department, hospitals, we are built for a twenty-four-hour day, every day. In an emergency, there is never a reason to wait for a better time to call us.

"We don't save the good staff for the daytime and punish the bad staff with night shifts."

While he doesn't recommend that anyone show up at 2 A.M. just to verify that the hospital is ready, Dr. Brown does encourage people to become informed about the health-care facilities in their area: "You really should know when you can visit your doctor's office, when you can visit clinics for nonemergency treatment. And you must understand that the time you can receive help for an emergency is anytime one happens."

Doctors tracked the outcomes of over 150,000 patients in critical condition based on the day of the week they arrived in the hospital. They found that patients' recovery rate did not vary based on whether they were admitted during the weekend or during the week. (University of Iowa 2002c)

A Relationship Starts with Yourself

People need loving human relationships. We all benefit from close social contact. But many of us think relationships will complete us—fill in any holes in our lives. In reality, if you are not happy with who you are, a relationship will not change that, and, in fact, it will be difficult for you to maintain healthy relationships.

TESS, A MIDDLE-AGED accountant from Toledo, Ohio, shares how her outlook has changed over time: "I used to see it as a chicken-and-egg problem. Which comes first: a healthy self-image, or healthy relationships? It seems like you need a healthy self-image to have healthy relationships, and you need healthy relationships to have a healthy self-image.

"Then I realized that I had less control over my relationships—people up and move on you, or they enter new phases of their lives without you—so that you have to start with yourself.

"If you don't think you are a good person, worthy of your own affection, it is hard for other people to disagree with you. On the other hand, when I really looked for the value in myself, it was easier for me to see it in other people."

In long-term studies of middle-class Americans, those who were satisfied with themselves and their lives ten years ago are today five times more likely to report having a happy relationship with a love interest. (Paris 1999)

Breathe Right

Proper breathing is probably the easiest and most powerful way to protect your health. It results in better digestion and circulation, more restful sleep, decreased anxiety, and a more stable heart rate.

FACED WITH MASSIVE road snarls during her daily commute, Julia, who lives in Atlanta, started reading up on breathing. She was surprised at the idea that something all of us do all the time could be improved so dramatically with a little thought and effort. Now, breathing right is her way of relieving stress while stuck in traffic.

"We all carry chronic tension in our lives," Julia says. "We don't even realize how much there is." Traffic jams can aggravate that tension and turn normally easygoing people into irritable road warriors, she adds.

"I know for myself, when I'm coming down the road and I see that traffic is backed up, that stress response automatically kicks in," she says. "Your heart rate speeds up, the muscles in your neck and arms begin to contract. Every muscle in your body is preparing for fight or flight. The problem is, you're not going to 'fight or flight.' You're stuck in traffic, and unless you do something right away, that stress response will stay in your body for hours or even days."

Julia's method is the one experts favor: "Take deep breaths. Let your abdomen rise like a balloon as you inhale, filling it all the way. As you exhale, let your abdomen gently relax back toward your spine."

Researchers found that breathing slowly and deeply from the abdomen triggers a boost in blood flow to the brain and up to a 65 percent reduction in stress. (Harvard University 2003)

Use Your Own Self-Interest

What is the difference between the most driven and the laziest person? Self-interest. We all do what we do because of self-interest: we think it's the best thing for us. Those who work hard do so because they believe there is a reward awaiting them that not only justifies their efforts but demands their dedication. Remind yourself of the value of the things you want, and the costs to you in effort will not feel as great.

GWEN GOT HER start training dogs and then soon realized her training was really of their owners.

"I would teach people about consistently reacting to what the dogs did so that good behavior was rewarded and bad behavior punished," Gwen says. "And I thought to myself, It's not the dogs that are being inconsistent here, it is the people.

"You have the gigglers who say 'Isn't that cute' when the puppy grabs their socks out of their hand and then get upset when the puppy goes for the sock, the shoes, the couch. You have the couples where one takes the strict approach and the other is in cahoots with the dog, covering up when the dog does something wrong.

"What dogs want is your love, attention, and treats. If you make it perfectly clear and consistent what it will take to get that reaction, your dog will behave because of self-interest. But it is also a matter of your self-interest," Gwen maintains. "If you are too lazy to be consistent with your dog, or if you really don't care what happens to your socks and shoes, then your lack of interest will come across."

Researchers find that perceived self-interest, the rewards one believes are at stake, is the most significant factor in predicting dedication and satisfaction toward work, accounting for about 75 percent of personal motivation toward accomplishment. (Dickinson 1999)

Doing Nothing Is Rarely a Solution

When we don't have an answer, it is tempting to ignore the problem. But you can ignore problems only so long until they grow far larger—and far harder to solve. Approach your relationship with all your attention and abilities, the way you would approach anything that is important to you.

"YOU MAY NOT find this on too many greeting cards, but the fact of the matter is arguing is pivotal to happy marriages," says Professor David Olson. "We know that all couples who marry are in love. Yet 50 percent of them divorce. And the biggest predictor of staying together is how well they're able to work through their differences."

Professor Olson says people need to understand that thoughtful love and careful conflict are two sides of the same coin. "Arguing well avoids the kind of scorched-earth disagreements that drain a relationship," he says.

Laurie and Dave took Professor Olsen's relationship questionnaire and received follow-up counseling. They credit his counseling with making their relationship stronger. She says she constantly avoided conflict in previous relationships. "This was a big issue in my first marriage," Laurie says. "We always had to have a winner and a loser. So I'd get scared of disagreements and basically run and hide from them."

She and Dave worked on that issue in sessions with a marriage and family therapist. "Dave help to reassure me there were other options than mega-arguments," Laurie says. Now, when Dave senses her withdrawing, he'll coax her to talk rather than clam up. "And I think we both help each other stay on track with whatever we're talking about—money, religion, whatever," Laurie says.

Married couples who report they never argue with each other are 35 percent more likely to divorce within four years than are those couples who report regularly disagreeing. (Vaughn 2001)

Accept Yourself—Unconditionally

Y̲ou are not just the size of your bank account, the neighborhood you live in, or the type of work you do. You are, just like everyone else, an almost inconceivably complicated mix of abilities and limitations.

A NEW KIND of New Year's resolution is becoming increasingly popular. Instead of dwelling on something they think is wrong with them and re-solving to improve, a lot of people are taking a different approach. They are resolving to accept themselves—to acknowledge that, faults and all, they are complete people, good people.

Kathleen, a member of a group that spreads the acceptance philoso-phy, explains that she used to feel like she was in a trap she could not get out of. She would try to correct herself and change herself, and the failure to change upset her more than the original problem itself. She felt like a "maniac" because of the pressures to change and the weight of failure.

Now Kathleen counsels accepting yourself, which does not mean ignoring your faults or never trying to improve. What it does mean, Kathleen says, is "believing in your own value first, last, and always."

Researchers have found that people who are happy with themselves take defeat and explain it away, treating it as an isolated incident that indicates nothing about their abilities. People who are unhappy take defeat and enlarge it, making it stand for who they are and using it to predict the out-come of future life events. (Brown and Dutton 1995)

Second-Hand Smoke Is Optional

Whether it is for a family member, a friend, or to be able to visit a favorite restaurant, many people would rather accept the burden of second-hand smoke than the costs of avoiding it. However, second-hand smoke is a serious and optional health risk. Think of it this way: you wouldn't accept a slap in the head just because other people felt like doing it.

MINNESOTANS HAVE WITNESSED a unique statewide advertising campaign about the dangers of second-hand smoke. The ads—which appear on television and the radio and in newspapers, on billboards, and in buses—were produced as part of a $5.5-million antismoking campaign funded by Minnesota's 1998 settlement with the tobacco companies.

"Second-hand smoke kills more Americans each year than murder, drugs, and AIDS combined," says Dr. Richard Hurt, chairman of the Minnesota Partnership for Action Against Tobacco.

Dr. Hurt notes that children exposed to second-hand smoke are more likely to have asthma, bronchitis, and pneumonia and to die of SIDS— sudden infant death syndrome. "Hundreds of thousands of children suffer needlessly because others smoke around them," Dr. Hurt says.

However, most Minnesotans "don't understand how serious a problem it is," he says. The ad blitz was designed to change that.

One thirty-second TV spot shows a dead bird in a cage with a cigarette burning underneath and the message "Second-hand smoke contains 200 poisons and 43 cancer-causing agents." All the ads end with the same tagline: "Second-hand smoke. Still want to breathe it?"

Children's exposure to second-hand smoke was found to be directly related to their mother's attitudes. The children of those who considered second-hand smoke unhealthy were 72 percent less likely to show exposure to second-hand smoke. (Columbus Children's Hospital 2002)

Listening Is More Than Not Talking

We think about what we have to say. How much to say. How best to say it. We invest so much thought in talking that we sometimes treat the time when we're not talking as a rest break. Instead, active listening, investing ourselves in what others are saying, is the only way we can learn from others and adapt what we have to say to correspond to the other person's perspective.

DON HAS BEEN married for forty-seven years.

He admits not everyone saw his potential for being a good husband. "My own mother used to wonder how my wife put up with me," Don says.

"If I ever told her about a disagreement we'd had," he adds, "she would tell me to turn right around and apologize. Every time.

"One time, while I wasn't paying very close attention, my wife told me an interesting story about a neighbor. The next day I repeated the story to her, forgetting that she had been the one who told me."

Before too long, Don says, he began to understand the importance of communication in their arguments: "We would argue about one person not doing what they agreed to do, or forgetting something important, and it became clear that the problem was we weren't paying enough attention in the first place.

"I realized that listening is a skill, and like any other skill, the less attention you give to it, the more mistakes you make. Only these are mistakes you can't cover up, because the person who was talking to you knows you made them."

Good talkers tend not to be good listeners. Good listeners are 60 percent more likely to try to put themselves in the other person's place—trying to see things through the speaker's perspective. (Pauk 1997)

You'll Get Knocked Down and Then Get Back Up

So many outcomes seem out of our control. Decisions are made that change our companies, our jobs, our lives, and yet we feel helpless to affect them. But if you can accept some uncertainty, and believe in yourself, there will always be alternatives available to you—you will always have a choice no matter what the situation.

AS HIS BROTHER was buried, another gang member killed in a gang war, William sat in his jail cell and cried.

And he found a purpose. Over the course of the next few months, another inmate taught him to read. Then William applied to take classes in prison to help him earn a high school degree, and after that he signed up for job training.

William's efforts earned him an early release. He immediately began looking for ways to help the next generation of young men avoid the kind of life both he and his brother had led. William set his sights on a program to bring children and police officers together, to forge positive relationships and bring role models into the children's lives.

"When I grew up, I looked up to the drug dealers, the big boys," William says. "They were the people who were tangible to me. When I look back at my brother's situation, at my situation, I see that a failure to see past that is what killed him."

When he's not working with children, William is back hitting the books. He's working on a degree in criminal justice, with an eye toward law school. "I think that'll reinforce my natural advocacy skills. I'd like to take my programs on a larger scale."

Self-image and acceptance of risk accounted for more than half of the reaction of those who faced significant change in the workplace and were more important than the actual changes themselves. (Judge et al. 1999)

Keep Your Fears in Line

A large part of our life is spent imagining the worst and its consequences. Step back from your fears and worries and realize that one of the biggest hurdles to overcome is not what you are afraid of but the fact that you are afraid.

"I GUESS I'M really the ultimate example of worrying yourself sick," says Marty.

Concerned about a persistent cough for which doctors could offer neither relief nor an explanation, Marty sought second, third, and fourth opinions.

A snowstorm had blanketed his town on the day he had an appointment for another opinion. Rather than reschedule, Marty insisted on clearing off his driveway and heading out to keep his appointment.

The combination of snow and ice made for tough going, and in an effort to gain some traction, Marty fell and landed on his arm. "Well, I was going to the doctor, there was no doubt about that. Only now I was thinking it might be an orthopedist instead," Marty says.

Marty had broken his arm. After a trip to the hospital, Marty returned in a cast.

With other things on his mind now, Marty canceled the appointment he was trying to get to in the first place. After a few weeks of rest, he found his cough gone but his arm very much still broken.

Marty has extracted two lessons from his experience. First, when it snows, stay inside. Second, worrying is more trouble than it's worth. "I think of it as kind of like that old saying 'Laugh and the whole world laughs with you. Cry, and I'll give you something to cry about.'"

Relative to their own doctors, most people were four times more likely to think themselves likely to suffer a debilitating illness in the near future. (Sarkisian et al. 2001)

Television and Eating Should Not Go Together

In many households, there is a constant guest for dinner: television. Television and eating complement each other, and encourage our overconsumption of both. It will help you develop sensible habits if you separate your television time from your eating time.

"I NOTICED IT affected not just what I ate but how much I ate," Debra says of watching television while she ate dinner with her son. "When you are watching television and eating, neither is your real focus. So you can just get lost in a program and not stop yourself from eating too much. Or get lost in eating and not stop yourself from watching too much TV."

And, she notes, "you'll eat anything, the worst things, with the television on. It's cookies and snacks and quick-fix meals." She compares it to hanging around with the wrong friends in school: "You'll do things you wouldn't otherwise do, and for no good reason."

When she decided to make a change, Debra not only cut down on what she ate and what she watched; she also eliminated the combination. "I have completely changed everything in my approach," she says, "and it really lets me appreciate more what I'm doing."

Each meal eaten in front of the television adds up to an hour devoted to daily television watching. (Cincinnati Children's Hospital 2002)

Think of Your Own Ideal

Think back to the first image you had of the person you imagined you would marry. The images come from things we were exposed to in the media, or perhaps our personal life. But, for many, it is hard to shake the relationship expectations that have surrounded us, even if their origins were in the ill-informed imagination of the child version of ourselves. We must move past the images from our youth or from fiction and forge a relationship around what truly matters to us today.

MICHELLE WAS SURE she had found the perfect man: "He had the right job, he had the right look, he had the right things. As far as I could tell, he was perfect." They married and started their life together in Philadelphia.

Then reality came in: "He became more remote with each passing day. It was as if I were married to a photo on the wall instead of to a person."

Michelle asked herself how this happened. Then, she says, "I thought about what I really knew when this started. He looked the part. And if I'd hired him to be an actor portraying my husband, I suppose it would have worked out all right."

Five years later, Michelle is happily in a relationship—this time, with someone she considers real. "I learned to pay attention to what matters," she says. "If you make a shallow decision based on what someone has to offer, money or looks, there's no reason to think they'll still have those things down the road. But if you find someone who has what really matters to you, a kind and generous spirit, they'll have that forever."

Research on marriages with high levels of conflict finds that more than half of the couples in these marriages have disputes involving the failure of one or both partners to conform to unspoken expectations. (Philpot 2001)

Communicate on Your Listeners' Terms

W hether it's a personal conversation or an important speech, the point of communication is to be understood. The desire to express ourselves in our own terms is strong and can lead us to lose sight of our audience. Don't think in terms of what you want to say; think in terms of what you want your listener to hear.

A ROOMFUL OF people sit silent and still. They are hanging on every word Jay has to say.

Jay is speaking just above a whisper, describing how a young woman slowly gains the trust of a ferocious tiger. One day the woman plucks one of the tiger's whiskers and scampers off to give the whisker to a wizard who needs it to concoct a potion.

The audience gasps and groans with each twist of Jay's story.

Jay is part of a growing community of people who practice the art of storytelling. "Sharing stories is a very humanizing part of life," Jay says.

Jay's stories are not read from a book, nor are his audiences limited to children. Jay tells stories as a way to offer entertainment and to feel a connection to an audience.

And when he's not telling stories, he offers a class on how to tell stories. Jay emphasizes the importance of the audience's perspective: "Storytelling requires sincere eye contact and natural hand gestures to really keep a listener's attention. You have to remember that holding their attention is the essence of the experience."

Jay believes that people have the potential to be much better communicators than they realize. "Many people have a great capacity for storytelling and don't even know it," Jay says.

People who said they thought about things from their listeners' perspective were 48 percent more likely to be rated as effective in their communication efforts. (Chen and King 2002)

Talk to Your Pharmacist

Pharmacists are often an overlooked resource in our health-care team. Pharmacists can help us understand the value and effects of different medications, help us follow the directions in taking them, and guide us to over-the-counter products that are safe to take in light of our particular condition. Speak to your pharmacist regularly, and you will dramatically reduce the chances of making a mistake with your medications.

LARRY'S MEDICATIONS CAME with a dizzying array of instructions: "Take with water." "Take with food." "Take as needed." "Take until empty." "Don't drive or operate heavy machinery after taking."

The statistics for using medication incorrectly are grim. Each year in the United States, one out of six hospital admissions, one out of four nursing-home admissions, half of medication failures—and 2.5 million medical emergencies—are attributable to incorrect medication use.

"People always have questions. They want reassurance and accurate information from somebody they can trust," says Professor Jerry Cable of Ohio State University.

Professor Cable's pharmacist outreach program helped answer these concerns. "We were looking for outdated medications, duplicates, and drugs that could interact with other drugs," Professor Cable says.

For Larry, the outreach program found two drugs that were meant to address the same problem. Larry was grateful for the information.

"People need someone to have oversight over their medications, because it is too important to ignore and too complicated for most people to fully understand," Professor Cable says.

Researchers found that people who took the opportunity to individually discuss their medical condition with a pharmacist wound up taking 13 percent fewer medications on a daily basis and had 60 percent fewer medication-related problems. (Ohio State University 2002)

Let Go of the Burden of Pain

You have to let go of the pain of being wronged. Carrying it around makes it seem like the hurt is fresh every day. Ask yourself this: if you had to walk one hundred miles and had the option of carrying a massive cement block, a block of no value to you or anyone else, or of carrying nothing at all, which would you choose? "Why would I possibly choose to carry this block?" you would say. Exactly.

BEFORE HE LEFT office, former President Bill Clinton said that he was focusing on "re-earning the trust and esteem of my family and the American people.

"While it is unusual for the president to be in a public situation like this, the fundamental truth is that the human condition—with its frailties and propensity to sin—is something I do share with others. And I believe in the reality of forgiveness.

"When you genuinely atone, and genuinely make the effort to change, that's an immensely liberating experience. It makes you stronger. It makes you straighter.

"Seeking forgiveness gives me a chance to make my marriage whole, and my relationship with all my other friends whole, in a way that the keeping of secrets that are destructive cannot. And I also believe the American people will be more likely to support me because every American has been broken by something in life.

"Each day should be a new beginning. I'm looking forward to tomorrow and all the tomorrows because I feel freer than I have in a long time."

Studies find that those who have experienced a significant disappointment from their partner and have successfully granted their forgiveness to their partner are as likely to maintain a satisfying relationship as are those who had never experienced a similar disappointment in their relationship. (Maltby, Day, and Barber 2005)

Boredom Is the Enemy

Boredom will eat away at your persistence and resolve. No one can do the same job, requiring the same tasks, with perpetual interest and enthusiasm. When evaluating a job opportunity, don't just worry about the salary and workload; investigate how much variety there is in the tasks you'll perform.

LOREN SCHULTZ HAS spent forty-five years running companies and riding the wave of technology in data management.

Some of his ideas have worked spectacularly well, and some have fizzled out, overtaken by something better.

"Everything we've done is based on someone having a new idea and pursuing it," Loren says.

He no longer starts companies from scratch, but uses his vast experience to run a business incubator, which provides office space, consulting, and capital to new businesses. What Loren loves is taking everything he's learned and using it to help newborn companies grow. "Every day is a different adventure," he says. "I'm like the grandfather around here: I'm not in charge of anything, but I'm available to talk about anything. I've got a lot of experience. Why not share it with people? And the best part of working with all these different companies is, it's fun."

Low job variety produces twice as much employee turnover as high job variety and three times less job satisfaction. (Melnarik 1999)

Share Housework

It's unpleasant. It's not fun. Nobody particularly enjoys it. But the burdens of housework must be shouldered. Relationships work best when both partners recognize these simple facts and embrace a sharing of the workload.

SUZANNE BIANCHI, A sociology professor, completed a major study of housework. She found that women shoulder the great majority of the burden. "We women have been brainwashed more than even we can imagine," she says. "Probably too many years of seeing media women in ecstasy over their shiny waxed floors or breaking down over their dirty shirt collars. Men have no such conditioning. They recognize the essential fact of housework ... Which is that it stinks."

She says that although neither men nor women want to do housework, women are more vulnerable to the situation: "If he begins to get bugged by the dirt and crap, he will say, 'This place sure is a sty' or 'How can anyone live like this?' and wait for your reaction. He knows that all women have a sore called 'guilt over a messy house.' If he rubs this sore long and hard enough, it'll bleed and you'll do the work. He can outwait you."

Professor Bianchi does see one important trend that may change this relationship. Notably, it's not men doing more work, but women doing less. "The path to equality, fortunately or unfortunately, goes through much less housework being done," she says. "In other words, you may not argue over who does the housework, but you'll be sitting on a pile of dust when you talk."

Couples who share housework duties report they are 19 percent more satisfied in their relationship than couples where one partner does the vast majority of the work. (Allen and Webster 2001)

Role Models Are Not One Size Fits All

We often see stories of inspiring people and wonderful successes. Some of us put their pictures on our walls or clip notable quotes from them. But what does that do for us if the inspiring person has done things we will never do, done things we could never do? For many of us, the choice of a role model invites comparison, and if our abilities and outcomes do not measure up, the role model serves not as an inspiration but as a source of frustration and defeat. Choose as your role model someone who has accomplished something you can accomplish and something you want to accomplish.

HEIDI MILLER HAS served as the chief financial officer for the multinational financial giant Citigroup, and later in the same position for the Internet sales business Priceline.com.

While she made her steady climb through the corporate world, each step brought her further into isolation.

Her old friends dismissed the corporate calling: "You're going to work for a bank, you're such a traitor," they'd say. Meanwhile, her colleagues were not terribly supportive. "I felt marginal," Heidi laments.

She knew that if she didn't receive the support she hoped for, there were many others like her going through the same experience. That's why she founded Women and Company, an association of businesswomen who meet periodically to share their exploits, offer support, and provide positive examples for each other. Heidi says she finds the group "fabulous because it is so reassuring."

People who actively target someone to serve as a role model draw positive feelings from that person only if the role model's achievements are both relevant and attainable. People who choose role models who do not fit that description wind up 22 percent less satisfied with their careers than people who do not have a role model at all. (Lockwood and Kunda 2000)

The Mirror Will Be Kinder

How we feel about our bodies has a lot to do with how we feel about ourselves. The good news is that we actually become more positive as we get older. We begin to see character where we once saw only flaws. We begin to see strength where we once saw only weakness. We begin to see ourselves where we once saw only the image we thought we should have.

IN 1999, A women's group in Rylstone, England, decided not to continue the traditional theme of its annual fund-raising calendar, which had always featured pictures of well-kept landscaped grounds. Instead, members of the women's group, ranging in age from forty-five to sixty-six, posed in the buff for the calendar.

Sales of the calendar, which every year the group hoped would bring in the equivalent of $2,000, instead made more than $1 million for leukemia charities.

Interestingly, the calendar sold well with both men and women. Women thought it was a tasteful and fun celebration of women's bodies. And men responded to the depiction of real women. As one man says, "How wonderful to see real women instead of stick insects with pouty lips and pipe cleaners for legs."

The calendar and its participants later inspired the film *Calendar Girls*.

As sociologist Ann Morgan argues, "Whether posing nude is a giant step forward is no doubt a whole other debate. But in claiming and proclaiming their bodies for themselves—and, by extension, others—these women have made a very positive gesture. The notion of a beautiful body image must be understood not for the exclusivity of beauty, but for its variety."

People become about 1 percent more likely to hold a positive image of their body for every year they are over the age of forty. (Reboussin et al. 2000)

Common Chores Can Be Dangerous

There are probably few things that seem less dramatic than guiding a lawn mower back and forth across a yard. But lawn mowers are capable of slicing not just grass, but nearly anything they come into contact with, including hands and feet. Never let a boring task distract you from the importance of safety.

MICHAEL McREYNOLDS WORKS hard to keep his yard in good shape and has spent more than his share of weekend afternoons mowing the lawn. But as a nurse with the Michigan-based Survival Flight program, which transports critically injured patients to the hospital, he's also seen devastating injuries that can come from mowing lawns.

"A lawn mower used carelessly is very dangerous," he warns. "But the vast majority of lawn-mower injuries are preventable."

One of the first things Michael does before he cuts the lawn is pick up loose debris on the lawn, especially since his children sometimes leave their toys around the yard. "Any clutter left lying around the yard can fly up into the engine and be projected out the side, almost like a missile, and it can cause serious injury," Michael says.

Personal protective equipment is also a must, according to Michael. To prevent injury, he suggests that everyone who operates a lawn mower wear pants, steel-toed boots, and goggles. In addition, Michael suggests using some form of hearing protection, since lawn mowers, at an average of 95 decibels, are extremely loud.

The single biggest danger, though, is the lawnmower blade. "You should never reach under a lawn mower for any reason. Even when the mower's turned off, the blade is still turning and there's still the risk of a severe injury," says Michael.

Researchers found that seventy-five thousand Americans are injured every year in lawn-mower accidents. (University of Michigan 2002c)

Foundations Are Created in the Beginning

Relationships are like the planets: they move, but they keep coming back to the same points. Relationships tend to orbit around their origins. If those origins are trust, love, and respect, then that will be the universe of that relationship. If those origins are something else, then the relationship is unlikely to ever be based on trust, love, and respect.

WHEN IT COMES to love, Shawn doesn't take any chances. Instead of entrusting her romantic destiny to Cupid's arrows, the twenty-eight-year-old from Tampa believes in a more scientific approach. Shawn has turned to textbooks, tests, and a marriage-preparation course to guide her two-year-relationship with her boyfriend.

"When we're on long car trips, I pull out my book and start discussing the chapters with him," she says. "At first he thought I was weird, but it has helped us examine the weaknesses in our relationship and to grow stronger.

"All this effort encourages self-evaluation of a situation. You may not be able to solve all your problems, but the books and the course could prevent you from making a mistake.

"The best part is that we've been creating healthy habits from the start," Shawn says. "Instead of letting a problem develop, and then having to try to undue some harm, we're trying to prevent problems and instill good communication. It's a lot easier to talk about something and head it off than it is to have to go back and undo something that has been going on."

Long-term studies of relationships find that the negative feelings expressed in the first year of a relationship strongly predict whether that relationship will continue on into the future, and whether it will be a happy relationship years later. (Huston et al. 2001)

Get Away from It All

In every life there should be regular moments of awe. For most of us, our homes and communities may meet our needs, but they seldom inspire us. Take time on a regular basis to put yourself in a completely natural setting. Leave the city, the suburbs, and see the forest and the trees.

CAROLE GREW UP on a busy street in the middle of Richmond, Virginia. "All day long, something would be happening," she says. Across the street was the bus depot—where all the buses returned at the end of the day and all the buses started up again at the beginning of the next day. As if that wasn't enough, there were her six siblings and all the attendant chaos.

When she was seven, her family took a trip out into Grayson County in the Virginia countryside. "It was like I landed on another planet," Carole remembers. "Everything was green, everything was alive, and beautiful, and the sky was so big, it looked like it went on forever. And, as far as you could see, no other people."

Carole never forgot that trip. Five decades later she returned to Grayson County and bought some land and a century-old house there. "We thought we were going to tear it down and build something new, but then I thought, 'This house belongs here,'" she says.

The house looks over a field and a glistening creek. "I like to listen to the creek. In fact, it's about the only sound out there most times," Carole says.

At first, she had to learn to sleep in such a quiet place. But the payoff was in the morning. "You wake up and the birds are singing. It's so peaceful," Carole says.

People who regularly experienced nature were 9 percent less likely to report feeling unsatisfied with their lives. (Gerdtham and Johannesson 2001)

Study Your Sports Drink

For exercise lasting forty-five minutes or less, there is no real advantage to drinking anything other than water. For particularly rigorous exercise, a sports drink might help you replenish yourself. You must study the labels, however, because some sports drinks are closer to junk food than nutrition.

TIM DUNN IS a doctor, and a weekend warrior in a local basketball league. He knows firsthand the dilemma facing active people when they reach for a beverage. "Drinks containing carbohydrates, protein, caffeine, herbal products, vitamins—all claim to be the perfect sports drink. So how can a person choose the right sports drink?" Dr. Dunn asks.

"There is no magic tonic that is going to make you jump higher, run faster, or transform you into an elite athlete," Dr. Dunn warns. "The purpose of sports drinks is to replace fluids lost during exercise."

He says the best source for fluid replacement is water: "It's what makes up most of our bodies. Water is abundant, inexpensive, and has been endorsed by Mother Nature for millions of years as the number one drink. Water should be our primary beverage for fluid replacement. However, during intense activities, or activities that last greater than forty-five minutes, water may not be enough."

But what should be in your sports drink?

According to Dr. Dunn, "the optimal sports drink should contain no more than 8 percent carbohydrates. Try to avoid sports drinks that are carbonated, contain caffeine or herbal remedies, and are greater than 8 percent sugar. Keep it simple."

Researchers have found that, for more than nine in ten people, water is the best beverage to drink for their typical exercise activity. Sports drinks are beneficial only for those athletes who participate in high-endurance activities. (Colorado State University 2002)

Make Change Count

W̱e are all tempted by change. Whether a change in procedure or a change in jobs, we are hit with a wave of enthusiasm as we focus on the potentially positive results.

All talented people want to make changes in their lives and in the world around them. If you believe you are talented, you begin with the notion that you can do things better and therefore you should.

But it makes no more sense to rush into every change you can effect than it would to run away from every change possible.

"I'VE TRIED TO go in so many directions, I don't know where I am anymore. I've tried so many programs, I've lost count," says Teresa, a paralegal in Charlotte, North Carolina. "Now I need a program for people who've tried too many programs.

"I fall for the sales pitch, I jump in, and then a short time later I don't feel like it's working. Then the cycle starts all over again.

"Finally, one of my friends told me that I have to approach changing my life more like I'm buying a house than like I'm buying a dress. It's not permanent and irreparable, but it ought to reflect serious consideration and a solid commitment.

"In a way, it's a good thing all these programs didn't work, because I've signed up for so many, I'd be fifty-six different people by now if they'd worked."

People who rate themselves as intelligent have a 47 percent higher need for change in their professional world. They regularly see possibilities and opportunities around them but must be wary of allowing boredom to encourage them to pursue change just for the sake of change. (Whatley 1998)

Develop a Healthy Calm

Maintaining your calm in stressful situations not only allows you to listen more closely to your partner but allows you to think more clearly about the situation. Although your inclination toward anger is in part a function of your personality, healthy habits such as eating fruits and vegetables and regularly exercising will lower your tendency toward lightning-quick anger.

"DO YOU KNOW that moment when you've said something, and just as the words are leaving your mouth you wish you hadn't said it? I used to have that happen to me all the time," admits Tom. "Unfortunately, thinking clearly is not required when you talk."

Tom was tired of the damage he was doing to his own relationship by saying things that exaggerated how he felt or were more hurtful than he had realized. Tom started reading up on communication skills, not just in relationships, but also in high-pressure and stressful occupations.

"I really began to see the dynamic at work. It was the 'You say something, I say something' contest. If you say something that knocks me back, I say something that knocks you back a little more. But what if you say something that knocks me back, and I don't say anything, I just think about it. Then I'm not as likely to come back at you and up the wattage of the argument," Tom says.

When he tried to implement his new communication strategy, "I didn't have any unrealistic expectations," Tom says. "I think things are better because I'm doing less damage in disagreements, which means I can try to help with solutions instead of making the problem bigger."

People who get angry quickly experience not only more arguments in their relationships, but arguments that continue 81 percent longer than do people who are prone to remain calm. (Berry and Worthington 2001)

Learn from Losses

The setbacks you experience are wonderful opportunities to learn. Not only can you learn what you might have done wrong, but you can gain understanding about what led you to make the choices you made. Are you pursuing the goal you truly want? Are you pursuing a goal whose steps you are suited for? Gain something every time things don't go your way.

IN COLLEGE, MARY Ann sweated through a pharmacy program, one of the most challenging majors available. She had her eye on a career that would pay well and perform a public service.

Only after graduating, she says, did she see the options that were truly available to pharmacists today: "Basically, you can sign on for life with a megapharmacy, work long hours in a windowless warehouse, slapping labels on bottles and never seeing, much less talking to, your customers. Or you can sign on for a small neighborhood operation that will either go out of business or be bought up by a superchain within six months."

Mary Ann opted for the megapharmacy and, not surprisingly, didn't enjoy her work.

After six years of very steady work, she and two colleagues began making plans to open their own store, where they could work on their own terms. "My desire for change overwhelmed my fears of what would happen out on our own," Mary Ann explains.

"I wasn't in the right place," Mary Ann says. "But I don't look at my decision as a disaster, because people often fail, but if they learn from failures, then they gained something in the process."

A majority of students who failed in college and later returned for their degree report that the biggest difference in their second chance was better knowledge of themselves and their capabilities and commitments. (Robeson 1998)

The Best Life Needs No Trophy

One of the challenges of pursuing a satisfying life is that there is simply no competition. You will never live a better life because of the failure of another, nor a worse life because of someone else's success. See your satisfaction on personal terms; it need not be justified to anyone or by anyone.

PAUL HAS BEEN swimming for more than seven decades. He's set records in his age group and won so many races that he's been inducted into the Swimming Hall of Fame. But he's never had more fun in the pool than with the swimming club he helped found.

"Most swimming clubs are focused on training for specific competitions. Everything is competitive. We wanted more from a club than training, exercise, and an occasional race," he says. "We wanted to create a friendly atmosphere for people who wanted to share their common love for swimming. Basically, we wanted to have fun, make friends, maintain good health, and improve as swimmers."

Doris has been swimming with the club for two years and can't tell you what her best time or her average time is. "Swimming with the club has helped me to improve my stroke, but I really don't care how fast anybody swims," Doris says. "I don't even care how fast I swim, even though I swim three to four miles a week. It is good for my circulation, and it makes me feel good."

"These are the greatest people in the world," Paul says. "My life is more fun now. That is what I wanted when we started, and I have it."

People who had above-average feelings of well-being were four times less likely to make frequent social comparisons, weighing their happiness and success against those of others. (Dube, Jodoin, and Kairouz 1998)

Control Your Health

The greater your sense of control over what you are doing and what will occur to you, the less wear and tear you will put on your body. By focusing on remedies and solutions to the problems that arise, you can keep your attention on what you can do in any situation instead of on what you can't.

WHEN HE DIDN'T get promoted, Dean fell into a negative spiral. He felt discombobulated. Out of sorts. "I was just sitting around. I couldn't focus on anything," Dean says.

With the disappointment at work came a challenge to his commitment to healthy eating and exercise habits. "I was basically saying to myself, 'Life is short. Maybe I should start enjoying myself," Dean says.

Nutritionist Ann Norris says life difficulties can overwhelm and undermine health goals: "Consumption of high-fat comfort foods can rise as much as 80 percent when people lose their job or have difficulties on the job.

"Something bad happens to them, and people may think losing weight right now or being healthy is insignificant in the scheme of things. But it can actually be even more important because it gives them something to focus on that they can control.

"Giving in to temptation will only heighten your sense that things are out of control. Putting limits on yourself, on the other hand, is a step toward feeling in control."

Researchers gave participants a skill test and exposed them to a loud, distracting sound. Those who were told the sound would go away if they succeeded on the test showed significantly fewer ill effects of the stressful situation than those who were told the sound would continue regardless of what they did. Researchers concluded that a sense of control calmed the first group, even though neither group really had any control over the process. (Pennsylvania State University 2002b)

Transitions Can Be Both Happy and Sad

We like to see things in clear terms: happy the opposite of sad. But our emotional life is more complicated than that. We can be happy and sad at the thought of transitions in our life. Understanding this allows us to see sadness not as the enemy of happiness but as a natural part of our reaction to our lives.

SHIVERING THROUGH A New York winter, Phil set out for Florida with visions of palm trees and sea breezes. He heard that the phone company was hiring, and put in an application. After hours of aptitude tests, he was hired and sent off to phone-installer classes.

"From the first day on the job I was comfortable with what I was doing. I liked it. I liked going out in a truck in the morning and being on the road and doing the work. I knew within a couple of days on the job that I would never want to do anything else," Phil says.

Over the years, the technology changed and the job got a bit more complex. "I liked the challenge. You had to learn something new every year," Phil says.

Thirty years later, Phil is retired. He takes care of the house and cooks for himself and his wife. He plays endless rounds of golf at a course that allows him to play free in exchange for his occasionally helping out with the grounds.

And how does it feel? "I feel like a kid again," he says. "Sometimes I'm the kid who just got out of school for the summer, and sometimes I'm the kid whose friends are all away at camp."

Researchers found that life events surrounding major life changes can produce strong feelings of both happiness and sadness at the same time. (Larsen, McGraw, and Cacioppo 2001)

Stay Safe in the Sun

Skin cancer is the most common form of cancer, occurring in more than 1 million Americans annually. Sun exposure and sunburn represent the leading preventable causes of skin cancer. Protect your skin when you're in the sun as you would protect yourself from any serious threat.

WHICH STATES' RESIDENTS are most likely to get sunburned? You would probably guess Florida or California or a state known for its sunny days. In fact, the highest rate of sunburn is found in states such as Colorado, Iowa, Michigan, Indiana, and Wyoming. "It seems to come down to sun-safe behaviors. The people in those states face fewer sun-oriented events such as beachgoing and may not be taking sun safety seriously," says dermatologist Timothy M. Johnson of the University of Michigan.

"While most people know that the sun's rays are dangerous, that does not always translate into action," says Dr. Johnson. "Practicing sun-safe behavior can protect against not only sunburn, but premature aging and the future development of skin cancer.

"But studies have shown that sunscreen users do not apply enough sunscreen to adequately protect the whole body."

The bottom-line advice from Dr. Johnson is this: "Use an SPF of at least 15. Use sunscreen any time you are going to be out in the sun for more than twenty minutes. Apply the sunscreen thirty minutes before you go outside. Pay a lot of attention to putting the sunscreen on your face, ears, hands, and arms, and reapply every two hours or immediately after swimming."

Surveys of more than 150,000 respondents found that 32 percent of Americans had been sunburned within the previous twelve months. Among those under eighteen, the rate was 80 percent. Exposure to sunburn triples the lifetime risk of skin cancer. (National Cancer Institute 2002)

Leadership Is Contagious

True leadership strengthens the followers. It is a process of teaching, setting an example, and empowering others. If you seek to lead, your ability will ultimately be measured in the successes of those around you.

"THIS ISN'T A job for individuals working alone, this is a job for a team," says police chief Frank Blane, who directs a department of one hundred officers in central California.

"I look at it as being a conductor of an orchestra, trying to make sure everyone is in tune," he adds.

Chief Blane sets the direction of the department in everything he does. "You have to be very, very fair to the officers," he says, "and then they get the message that they have to be that way to every citizen they interact with.

"The way chiefs get in trouble is showing favoritism. When the top goes bad, then the rest of the organization goes bad. But when the top sets the right tone, then everybody can follow that lead."

Despite the power we associate with the idea of a leader, 93 percent of those who actually lead an organization view themselves at least partially as a servant of the people in their organization. (Boyer 1999)

Don't Romanticize the Past

In many respects, we are prone to having positive notions of the past: times were simpler, life was easier, families were stronger. While we face challenges in finding and keeping relationships today, we also see the opportunities and the freedom available to us that were nonexistent in the past.

MICKEY ROONEY IS a living piece of show-business history, having performed from childhood past an age when most people would be long retired.

He still performs a variety act around the country. The show is a retrospective of his career and his life. He is joined (live) onstage by his wife, Jan Chamberlin Rooney. And via film clips of movies and shows that are shown to the audience during the performance, he's joined by many of his seven previous wives.

While the temptation to be melancholy about his personal life is great, Rooney takes delight in celebrating his life and loves. He admits to the audience that his life was empty before he married his first wife, Ava Gardner. He then adds, "Married life with Ava was great. Boy could she cook. Ever had fried water?"

As he pokes fun at the checkered course of his relationships ("I've been married so many times, I've got rice marks on my face"; "Alimony is like pumping gas into someone else's car. I've pumped a lot of gas"), he also dedicates the show to Jan Chamberlin Rooney. At the end of the show, Jan and Mickey sing "Let's Call the Whole Thing Off" before he sheepishly asks her if she'll put up with him for one more day.

Studies comparing relationships today to relationships fifty or more years ago find that levels of commitment are largely unchanged and that the biggest difference is that freedom of choice to enter and maintain relationships was less prevalent then. (Medora et al. 2002)

Laughter Really Is Medicine

Laughter helps us deal with pain and with difficulties and is valuable in a medical context because it reduces our anxiety and our body's state of alarm. Take time out when you are sick or worried about your health to watch your favorite comedy or read your favorite amusing book.

DR. STEVE ALLEN JR. is a family physician and medical professor at the State University of New York. He has lectured for two decades about the role of humor in healing. He is the son of the late actor and humorist Steve Allen.

Dr. Allen has been known to tell jokes and juggle to help calm his patients or even when he is presenting information to other doctors. Dr. Allen says that laughter has both health benefits and life benefits: "It helps people learn better, become more creative and resolve conflicts. And it makes people feel a lot better."

Research backs up Dr. Allen's beliefs.

Steven Sultanoff, former president of the Association for Applied and Therapeutic Humor, says studies show that laughter seems to increase antibodies that fight upper-respiratory diseases and other infections. It reduces stress by lowering serum cortisol, which the body releases under stress. Humor also increases tolerance to pain, which is why Dr. Sultanoff always listens to a funny tape when he drives to the dentist.

"We know the way we think is directly related to the way we feel," Dr. Sultanoff says. "People can think themselves into being depressed, anxious, or angry. But with humor, we shift negative thinking, and it becomes positive thinking."

Researchers found that people who laughed the least were 40 percent more likely to suffer from heart disease than people who laughed most frequently. (University of Maryland-Baltimore County 2002)

View Your Life As a Choice

In some sense, everything that has ever happened to you reflects the collective results of an almost infinite series of choices. From the trivial to the crucial, your choices brought you to this moment. Recognizing that your choices matter gives you the opportunity to accept the situations you encounter and to decide the future you want.

PART OF THE year it was much too cold. And part of the year it was much too hot. But Tom treated each day delivering the mail in the same Indianapolis neighborhood as a chance to do work he enjoyed, surrounded by people he liked.

Tom made friends with residents as he delivered the pieces of paper that defined their lives: wedding announcements, college acceptances, job offers, and love letters. He went to their parties and their funerals. He cherished his job for its simplicity, the friendliness, and the routine and rhythms of his days.

Over the course of his career, Tom had many opportunities to switch to a different route. He could have had one with less walking or less climbing. But he always declined, because he didn't want to leave the neighborhood he felt so close to. "A lot of the people have gone through pretty much every stage of my life as it developed over the years," Tom says.

Tom's co-workers have long admired his attitude. "He said, 'This is the work I chose.' He never complained," one says. "He loves getting up at the crack of dawn, because he is going to get out there and he is appreciated."

People who said they had significant disappointments in the outcome of their lives were 14 percent less likely to dwell on those disappointments if they viewed the outcome as a reflection of their choices and not as something they were powerless over. (Robinson-Rowe 2002)

Life Is Not a Zero-Sum Game

Your time is not literally an accounting of minutes. Though your budget is an accounting of dollars, your time is a measure of commitment, concern, and efficiency in addition to quantity. You can do more because you can use your time better. Take out a few frivolous time killers and work harder at using time well. By doing this, you can add to both sides of your life's equation.

"MY FATHER GAVE me a book of lawyer jokes. I've heard them all," says Michigan attorney Douglas Theodoroff.

"Sometimes lawyers get a bad rap, but we probably deserve it," he adds.

But Douglas is known as one of the good guys, a lawyer who takes time out from his thriving practice to donate it to clients who cannot afford to pay. "I almost consider myself a legal social worker. I enjoy solving problems for people. I have something I can share. If I can help people less fortunate, I want to do it," Douglas says.

Douglas says that even though he has a heavy workload, it's never overwhelming, because he imposes some order over it. "As you get older, it's easier to establish your priorities and not feel pressured to take on every paying client available," he explains.

Douglas also serves his clients' interests and his own time demands by trying to find solutions out of the courtroom. "Going to court is the most expensive and time-consuming outcome. It should be a last resort," he says.

The quantity of hours spent working or thinking about work, or hours spent with our families, does not predict achievement or satisfaction. Instead, the quality of those hours, how stressful or relaxing they are, is a much more potent factor in producing both a satisfying family life and career. (Brown 1999)

Don't Confuse Stuff with Success

You are neither a better nor a worse person for the kind of car you drive, the size of your home, or the performance of your mutual funds. Remember what really matters in your life.

DANNY TARTABULL WAS one of the most feared sluggers in baseball in the late 1980s and early 1990s. In 1992, he signed with the New York Yankees with what was then one of the richest contracts in major league baseball history.

Tartabull enjoyed the life of a superstar in New York, even appearing as himself on an episode of *Seinfeld*. When his playing career ended in 1997, Tartabull kept the lifestyle of a highly paid athlete.

He lived in huge homes with picturesque views. He leased a series of homes in Florida for which he paid more than $16,000 per month in rent. The only problem was that he didn't have the salary to support the lifestyle.

Newspapers began reporting that he had been evicted, then evicted again, then sued for hundreds of thousands of dollars in overdue rent.

"The lesson here," says one teammate who knew Tartabull before he played for the Yankees, "is that you can't live like you're going to be a baseball player your whole life."

The availability of material resources is nine times less important to happiness than the availability of "personal" resources such as friends and family. (Diener and Fujita 1995)

Respond to Stress

Stress is an accumulation of events and circumstances that represent more than we can handle. Stress eats away at our ability to function, both mentally and physically. The best response to stress is to not push yourself and wait for it to go away. Stress can be reduced, not only by avoiding the circumstances that are causing it, but by allowing for healthier outlets for your pressures.

RUBY HAS BEEN running a flight school, teaching people how to fly small airplanes, for forty-six years. It's quite a feat. Even more so when you realize she didn't start until she was in her forties.

Ruby oversees all aspects of the flight school, from accounting to maintenance to schedules. "I'll never retire," Ruby says. "I enjoy my work too much. And I haven't found any of it hard."

When she got her pilot's license, there weren't a lot of women in the air. "It just wasn't something women were expected to do. You got a lot of strange looks from the other pilots," Ruby says.

Still, she loved flying. "It's hard to explain why it's so much fun," she says about flying. "You're up there by yourself, and it's quiet and peaceful. On a stressful day I could just go up in the air. It clears everything up. It's relaxing.

"It becomes second nature. It's a beautiful thing, a totally different world."

While she's long since given up piloting, she says she still gets a thrill from watching the next generation learn how to fly: "It's like they are taking me up there with them."

People over age fifty were two times less likely to be proactive in response to periods of high stress in their lives than were people under age forty. (Simons 2002)

Have an Orange

Vitamin C, found in many fruits, including oranges, inhibits the process of artery clogging and lowers blood pressure. Regular consumption of vitamin C has been found to reduce the risk of heart attack, stroke, and premature death.

JOHN WAS RAISED on a citrus farm in Southwest Texas. He remembers the best and the worst of the farming experience, from the bumper crops to the crop-scorching droughts.

The farm had been in his family for generations, but when it was time for him to choose a career, he decided to leave the farm and become a teacher. At school, he would use the farm as an example in all sorts of lessons, from math to science. "There was so much that could be learned from the example," John says. He also reminded his students to eat oranges—just about the healthiest food he could think of.

While his father continued to run the farm, John helped out when he could. Then the worst disaster that can befall a citrus farmer struck—a freeze. A rare cold snap came through and killed all the trees. John's father was heartbroken and decided to retire from the farming business.

While worried over what would become of the farm, John was not ready to give up teaching. He decided to do both. "I'm doing two things I value. In different ways, both contribute to people's lives and help meet their basic needs," he says.

Each ounce of vitamin C–laden fruits consumed per day reduces the risk of premature death by 10 percent. (Cambridge University 2002)

Share the Praise and Share in the Blame

A relationship is a team effort. Neither the credit for a good day nor the blame for a bad one belongs entirely to one person. Openly sharing in both the credit and the blame, however, strengthens the team.

"I'LL TELL YOU my relationship philosophy," says George. "It comes down to two phrases: 'I'm sorry' and 'Thank you.' If you overuse those two phrases, things will go smoothly."

People keep asking George for answers because he's been married over sixty years. "I love my wife and always have. We enjoy being together. It's a recognition of being proud of somebody. You're willing to help them to make them happy," he says. "We've never fallen out of love, and we do things together. We would never think of divorce. We're probably a one-in-a-million couple. I would never think of living with anyone but my wife. She's a sweetie."

But George and his wife, like many other couples who married when they did, faced tough challenges. He says their commitment toward each other made it easier to surmount those challenges, though: "Because it was so easy being married, we could better handle the hard times when others were turning against each other because it was so easy to do."

Because money was scarce, George's first Valentine's Day gift to his wife was a stick of gum. "And you know what? She says it was the best gum she'd ever had," George says.

In interviews about their relationships, people were three times more likely to emphasize the role of their partner in problems and twice as likely to emphasize the role of themselves in strengths of their relationship. (Johnson et al. 2001)

Embrace Work—It May Have to Last Forever

We live in a culture that cherishes the dream of early success followed by early retirement. We read of a retirement utopia awaiting those who can afford it. In truth, most retirees base their identities on their careers and yearn for the activity and responsibility their work lives provided.

FOR EIGHTY-ONE-YEAR-OLD Vincent, a lifelong New York resident, retirement after sixty years of work has not been a dream come true. "Some people seem so happy to be retired, but I feel lost. A sense of fulfillment is missing," Vincent says.

But by serving on the local community board, which makes decisions on zoning and land use, he has found a way to keep himself engaged. "The community board keeps me moving," Vincent says.

The board, which is unpaid, often has to deal with contentious disagreements pitting neighbor against neighbor. Vincent says he tries to keep everyone calm, and to keep his comments to a minimum: "If I say something, it has to be worth saying." But when the time comes to take a vote, he calls on a lifetime of experience. "I've run more organizations than I now have hairs on my head. I think, 'What did I do then?' That helps," Vincent says.

The single biggest factor in shaping a retired person's identity is their career history, outweighing even their family life. (Szinovacz and DeViney 1999)

Don't Gamble Your Future

In the ads, everyone who places a bet or buys a lottery ticket is a winner. In reality, all forms of gambling are based on the inevitability of loss. Gambling can make us feel out of control, not only over the outcome of a wager, but of our lives.

SUSAN GAINES CONDUCTS research on gambling and people who gamble. She says the picture of the problem gambler is changing rapidly to include more women and more people middle-aged and older. And the reason, she says, is clear.

"It's a process that starts with scratch-off lottery tickets and bingo and then progresses to slot machines."

Susan says that growth within the gambling industry largely depends on finding new customers: "Casinos work hard to offer some characteristics very important for individuals who in the past would not gamble," she says. Slot machines and other electronic gambling devices offer what Susan says is a welcoming environment to the novice gambler, and to women in particular: "It's relatively cheap way to begin playing; it feels physically safe and attractive. For a lot of people, it's an antidote to boredom.

"New gamblers don't like to be aggressive or carry on a conversation with a blackjack dealer," says Susan. "They want to get off by themselves, be safe, and sit down with nobody bothering them. It's real easy for someone to get sucked in to slot machines. They're mesmerizing. You lose all consciousness of the value of money.

"Nobody chooses to develop a gambling problem, of course. But you need to watch out, especially if you begin to shield others from your gambling plans. It's the first step toward losing control."

Adults over sixty who regularly gamble are 17 percent less likely to feel satisfied with their lives and 9 percent more likely to feel their lives are not within their control. (Winslow 2001)

Combinations Matter

There are many medications that are safe and effective when taken alone but ineffective or counterproductive when taken in combination with something else. When taking over-the-counter medications, remember that the effects of a drug must be understood in light of everything else you are taking. Always using the same pharmacy will make it easier for the pharmacist to track all the medications you are taking and alert you if any might counteract each other.

A SURVEY BY the National Consumers League found that almost half of the people questioned said they had knowingly exceeded the recommended dose of over-the-counter pain relievers. Fewer than 20 percent said they had read the label completely.

Millions who take over-the-counter painkillers every year are unaware of their potential hazards. As a result, experts say, many people misuse these enormously popular drugs, which are used to treat a multitude of ailments including headaches, arthritis, viruses, and muscle pain.

The problem is that many Americans take the aggressively marketed pills thoughtlessly, "popping these things like they're candy," in the words of liver specialist Dr. William Lee.

Dr. Lee points to a popular flu-relief medication that warns patients not to take more than four doses in a twenty-four-hour period: "What it doesn't say is that just as dangerous as taking a fifth dose would be to combine the flu medicine with any number of popular pain relievers. And that's what we see far too much of: products which warn you what not to do with that product in particular, but which ignore the strong possibility that you might be taking something else at the same time."

People who take aspirin regularly to help prevent heart attacks may void its effectiveness by regularly taking other common pain relievers such as ibuprofen. (University of Iowa 2002a)

Resolve to Pursue Resolution

Do you feel like you've had this argument before? The ability to maintain some flexibility in both your ideas and your habits will decrease your inclination to disagree and increase your ability to compromise and move toward a solution.

A TEAM OF professors from the United States and Great Britain recently concluded that "masculinity is in a real moment of transition."

What that means is that the behavior of young men, and the preferences of young women, are evolving. "I was really struck by the younger people's ideas," Professor Jane Pollins says, "because they are responding to incredibly sensitive men who have real skills in conflict resolution. These men are very different from the kind of tough, macho men who were once seen as the ideal," she says.

She sees younger generations of men as evolving differently from their fathers and grandfathers. According to Professor Pollins, "men may have found a new emotional literacy, one that contradicts the traditional masculine stereotype but nevertheless is the man of the moment—sporting hero, style icon, and family man all rolled into one."

What interests Professor Pollins is that "this can create a supportive emotional relationship. Men who come into relationships with this kind of personal outlook tend to maintain it and bring forward healthier communication patterns for years to come."

Marital satisfaction is dependent on conflict resolution styles—the means by which both parties attempt to resolve disagreements. For 85 percent of marriages, those styles became set for both parties in the first year of marriage. Change was possible, but only when people became aware of their rigid tendencies. (Schneewind and Gerhard 2002)

Limit Your Exposure to Pesticides

There is a more important consideration than how green your lawn is, how vibrant your flowers are, or how big your vegetables are. And that is how much harm the pesticides you use are causing. You use pesticides in your garden because they are deadly to insects and other threats. But their power is also their weakness. Too much exposure to pesticides is not only a threat to pests but a threat to humans, pets, and other creatures. Consider natural alternatives to pesticides.

ROBINA WAS DROPPING her sons off at school one sunny spring day in Los Angeles when she saw a man wearing a hazardous-materials suit spraying the side of the building. Her sons walked right into a fine mist of what turned out to be pesticide. Her younger son, who had asthma, immediately experienced a severe respiratory attack.

Robina did research and found out that school maintenance workers were spraying pesticides and herbicides at levels ten times higher than the manufacturer's recommended strength.

Since then, Robina has founded a nationally recognized program in the Los Angeles Unified School District that alerts parents to the use of chemical sprays on school campuses, allowing parents to make alternate arrangements to address their children's needs.

The National School Pesticide Reform Coalition released a report highlighting the school district's policy as one of twenty-seven exemplary programs around the country. Robina was honored by Environment California for her efforts.

"It's been an effort of love in terms of protecting kids," says Robina, who spends many of her weekends at health fairs to spread the word about pesticides. "I want to help other people so their kids don't get sick."

A study found that those who frequently used pesticides at home had a 70 percent higher risk of getting Parkinson's disease. (Emory University 2002b)

Even in a Relationship,
You Are Still an Individual

Typically we do not find *one couple* pursuing one purpose in a relationship. We find *two people* in a relationship, each pursuing individual dreams. The strongest relationships support both partners' dreams, even if they differ—not one partner's dreams at the expense of the other's.

LANA AND DEREK moved in together seven years ago for practical reasons. Derek's lease was up, and his building was being turned into condominiums. "I think we would have done it anyway," Lana says. "That kind of maybe prompted it a little."

They had being seeing each other for a year, but before they moved in together they sat down and carefully discussed how money and household duties would be handled. Thus far their system has worked well: they split everything fifty-fifty.

Lana says that the issues that come up during their relationship are probably the same as those in any other relationship: "We try very hard to strike a balance between being together and letting both of us individually be the person we want to be. I work for a large company, and I'm a bit of a workaholic; he's an artist. So at times we're both on our own, running around doing the things that make us tick. But we both understand that our work can only bring us so far and that sharing with each other makes it all more worthwhile.

"We have a strong commitment to each other, which I think will last because we also have a strong commitment to ourselves. Because I think that's what makes a relationship commitment sustainable."

Eighty-eight percent of people surveyed reported that maintaining their sense of independence and equality was an important factor in their relationship decisions. (Thornton and Young-DeMarco 2001)

Want Support? Deserve It

When someone in the office gets promoted, will colleagues offer support and sincere congratulations, or will they snipe and complain? The difference comes down to whether they think the promotion was deserved. Which means, to maintain the support of your co-workers as you advance, you have to let them see how hard you are working long before the promotion as well as after it. You have to let them see how capable and dedicated you are.

STERLING AND SHANNON Sharpe grew up playing football together on the family farm in Glenville, Georgia.

Sterling, the older brother, was recruited by a football powerhouse, the University of South Carolina, and went on to become a first-round draft pick in the National Football League. Shannon was not heavily recruited and wound up playing football in obscurity at Savannah State College before fighting his way onto an NFL roster as the last man drafted by the Denver Broncos in 1990.

Sterling was among the league's best wide receivers, trying desperately to help his team to the Super Bowl, when a neck injury cut short his career. Shannon's skills continued to develop, until he too became recognized, as one of the premier pass catchers in the game.

Shannon's Denver Broncos made it to two consecutive Super Bowls. Then he won a third Super Bowl as a member of the Baltimore Ravens. When Sterling was asked whether he was jealous of his brother's continued success and Super Bowl rings, he said, "It's very easy to pull for him, because I know what this means for him and I know how hard he worked to get there."

Over eight in ten people will support their friends moving up beyond them, even support the advancement of peers with whom they are not friendly, if they feel the promotion was based on achievements and ability. (Feather 1999)

Make "Should" and "Want" the Same Thing

In the competition between "should" and "want," "want" often wins even though in the long run it may not be good for us. The way past this problem is not to try to constantly deny yourself the things you want, but to increase your appreciation for what you should do. Over time, you can increase your life satisfaction by increasing the balance between shoulds and wants.

KATIE THINKS IT'S the hardest question in family life: "When do I come first? I know it's not always. But it shouldn't be never, right?" With four children and a husband, she sometimes feels she's just an extension of their needs. "It seems you'll never eat a meal when it's hot, never finish reading an article, never finish flossing before the next request comes in," Katie says.

She considered but rejected starting what she calls a "blanket 'Find it yourself, fix it yourself, do it yourself' rule."

In her search for an answer, Katie says, she "started to look at things from the perspective of the entire family. It's not about what's convenient for me or for my husband or children. It's about what's good for the family."

Katie says, "The best answer requires you to look at things differently. What I want and what my family wants is not really the point. What they need, what I need, and what we all should be doing is the only thing that matters." And now, Katie says, she doesn't mind the requests as much, but "I only stop flossing for emergencies."

People who feel there is a difference between what they *should* do for a family member and what they *want* to do are 15 percent less likely to feel satisfied with their family life than people who think what they should do and want to do are the same thing. (Janoff-Bulman and Leggatt 2002)

The Fun Is Not Over

Fun is for young people. They have the time, they have the opportunity, they have the ability. Those may be common assumptions, but none are true. Though the source of fun and happiness may change over the course of life, there is no reduction in our ability or desire to have fun as we age.

SEVENTY-FOUR-YEAR-OLD Jack McKeon has spent nearly all his adult life involved in major league baseball. He has run teams from the dugout and from the front office.

In 2003 he was out of baseball. "I wasn't retired," he says, "just in between jobs." Then, the Florida Marlins called, two months into the baseball season. They needed a new manager who could turn the team's fortunes around. Immediately.

With no hesitation, McKeon took the job, becoming the third-oldest manager in baseball history. He found himself surrounded by ballplayers younger than his grandchildren. But he had no fear that he could no longer relate to young players. "Being around these guys has made me a young kid again," Jack says. "I feel so young I quit using my senior-citizen discount at restaurants."

Jack still has a serious competitiveness that motivates him to show up at the stadium ten hours before a game. And he expects his players to share that drive. But he never lets himself or his players forget that "baseball should be fun." He says, "If you are happy and relaxed, you thrive. If you are a tense perfectionist, this game will break you down."

Jack's team hardly broke down as he led the Marlins to a World Series victory in 2003.

In studies of people over fifty, each additional fun activity engaged in per month increased the likelihood of life satisfaction by 2 percent. (Cameron 1972)

Build Your Energy Level Gradually

If you get tired easily, remember that you weren't always tired all the time. Whether an underlying medical condition or an overwhelmingly busy life brings on fatigue, practical strategies can eventually improve your energy level. But improvement will not be as easy as flipping a switch. Endurance is built slowly, over time.

"FATIGUE IS A symptom that challenges doctors. It is hard to define, because it can feel different for each individual," says Dr. John Francis. "Fatigue is perplexing because it can accompany many different physical ailments, and it can also be related to anxiety, depression, not enough sleep, too much sleep, lack of exercise, too much exercise, or stress."

Dr. Francis says that a physician will usually proceed like a detective, getting as much information about the symptoms and medical history as possible and then following leads and exploring possibilities.

Dr. Francis offers his patients three steps toward greater energy, all of them focused on moderation and building slowly toward an improvement. "You should exercise, but do it gradually. Start slowly, so you don't increase your fatigue, and try to build up to twenty to thirty minutes of activity per day. You should seek to set a manageable and even pace in your work and daily activities. In other words, set priorities, and manage your time and energy efficiently. And you should practice good sleep habits. Establish a ritual for going to bed. Don't take work to bed, don't consume too much caffeine from coffee, teas, colas, and chocolate, and maintain a firm time for going to bed and waking up. Then, step-by-step, you can improve your energy level."

Among those who complained of frequent fatigue, immediate health improvements were rarely seen, but gradual lifestyle changes improved energy levels for nine in ten study participants. (University of Minnesota 2002b)

Meaningful Commitment
Is Mutual Commitment

Increasing your commitment to your relationship will not help unless you do so with your partner. On a rowing team, everybody has to try hard, but no one can try harder than anyone else; otherwise, the boat goes in circles. The same is true in a relationship.

DRS. JOHNNY AND Peggy Emberson of Georgia gave up their practices. His was obstetrics and gynecology, and hers dental. Instead of continuing lucrative careers in the United States, they headed off for Nepal, where they would donate their skills as medical missionaries.

"You always get more than you give," says Johnny of donating one's time and effort. Peggy says she and her husband just want to use their gifts to the best of their ability.

Peggy says only a very small percentage of the population of Nepal has medical care and that the country has a high infant mortality rate. The Embersons work out of a hospital in Kathmandu, the capital city, and also help train workers in rural areas.

How did they make such a momentous decision to give up not only practicing medicine in the United States but living here? "We are equal partners in everything we do," Peggy says. "It is how we started together, and it is how we continue together. Johnny put me through dental school; then I put him through medical school. We were partners on this decision 100 percent. One person can't very well decide to send a couple to Nepal, but because we're on equal footing, we can both make a sacrifice for each other, and for a greater good, and feel right about it."

In studies of the health of relationships over time, the most stable and successful relationships did not feature the highest level of total commitment from partners but close to equal levels of commitment from each partner. (Drigotas, Rusbult, and Verette 1999)

You Will Give Up Faster If You're Not in Control

Some people will give up the moment an obstacle is placed in front of them. Some people will doggedly continue to pursue a goal even after years of frustration and failure. Those who persevere recognize that they are ultimately responsible, not just for pursuing their goals, but for setting them. When you are in control, what you do matters, and giving up will not seem very attractive.

DARNELL ELLIS, A blues guitar man, once played alongside musical legend B. B. King.

Then alcohol addiction brought on a series of troubles in his life. When circulatory problems in his legs forced him to seek medical attention, he ran out of money—and hope. Evicted from his apartment while in the hospital, he returned to find that all his possessions, including his guitar, had been sold by the landlord.

He lost his home, his friends, and his career, and fell into depression.

Social workers who helped Darnell get off the streets had trouble lifting his spirits. Then they realized how important it was to help Darnell get a guitar.

"I had given up and lost the will, until I got the guitar." Darnell explains. "When people play an instrument, they feel in control. The world is on a string, and it's just the way you want it to be."

With his guitar in his hand, Darnell has hope. "At the end of each tunnel, there's a light. And you know something? I may not walk so fast, but I'm walking. So I'm on my way," Darnell says.

Research comparing students of similar ability found that the feature that distinguishes those who maintain a strong work ethic in their studies from those who give up is a sense of control. Those who expressed a sense of control received significantly higher grades than those who do not. (Mendoza 1999)

Anything Beats Boredom

There is only one true waste of time: boredom. Boredom is feeling that there is nothing worth doing. Your time becomes a hurdle to overcome instead of a resource to treasure. Doing absolutely anything is more productive than boredom.

"WHAT'S THE EXPRESSION," Harold asked, "about how something boring is about as exciting as watching paint dry? Well, I'll tell you, there were days I would have signed on for that in a minute. 'Which wall will be dry first?' I'd wonder. 'It looks dry on top, but I bet you can't touch it yet.'"

Harold took early retirement from a career in the construction industry with the idea that he could do all the things he'd ever wanted to do but never had the chance to do. "But then after I did all the things I'd always wanted to do, I was lost," Harold says.

Harold didn't really want a job, but when a friend suggested there were other ways he could put his knowledge and background to good use, it led him to his local planning and zoning committee. The committee advises the city council on proposed new construction projects, whether they are appropriate for the town and whether the plans fit the character of the neighborhood involved. Harold was appointed to a seat on the committee and found himself fascinated by the task. "You really see the town on another level from this vantage point—and it always gives me something to think about," he says.

People who frequently experienced feelings of boredom were three times more likely to describe their lives as empty and two times more likely to be apathetic about their future. (Bargdill 2000)

Most People Are Sensitive to Whitening Teeth

A word of caution to those who want to brighten their smile by whitening their teeth. Many people will feel an uncomfortable sensitivity after using at-home whitening products. Consult your dentist to determine whether whitening is appropriate, especially if you have fillings, crowns, or receding gums.

THE DESIRE FOR bright smiles is the latest trend in cosmetic dentistry that's sweeping the country. In fact, tooth whitening is the most requested cosmetic dental procedure according to the American Academy of Cosmetic Dentistry.

Besides that, new over-the-counter products—whitening strips, paint-on gels, toothpastes—seem to hit the market every week, boosting annual sales of the tooth-whitening industry into the billions of dollars.

There are important differences between whitening procedures performed by a dentist and those you can do at home. In-office bleaching procedures using either hydrogen peroxide or carbamide peroxide, for example, typically cost $350 to $600, while custom-made teeth trays prepared by a dentist for home use run about half that. Over-the-counter products, which contain solutions with weaker peroxide concentrations than those dispensed by dentists, cost between $15 and $40.

"For folks who just want to dabble with whitening, these store-purchased kits can work, but they're not as effective—or as strong—as what patients can get in a dental office," Dr. Christian Kammer says. Inappropriate use of over-the-counter bleaching products also can cause significant damage to tooth enamel, the Wisconsin dentist warns.

After one week of at-home whitening treatments, 54 percent of patients reported mild tooth sensitivity, 8 percent reported moderate sensitivity, and 4 percent reported severe sensitivity. (University of Southern California 2002)

Like the Way You Look

I f you are not comfortable with your image of your body, you will not be comfortable with anyone else's image of your body. And if that happens, it will erode your self-confidence and will make it much more difficult for you to find or maintain a relationship.

ANYONE WHO'S EVER had a bad-hair day knows how it undermines self-confidence. Now a psychology professor's research confirms this.

"Bad-hair days affect self-esteem, increasing self-doubt, intensifying social insecurities, and making people more self-critical in general," says Professor Marianne LaFrance.

And bad-hair days affect men, too, her study found: troubled hair makes women feel more disgraced, embarrassed, ashamed, or self-conscious, while men feel more nervous, less confident, and more inclined to be unsociable.

The study, which had an ethnically diverse group of young people fill out psychological tests, found that just the thought of a bad-hair day caused both men and women to feel they were not as smart as others.

Professor LaFrance warns, "We talk about self-esteem coming from the inside, but the reality is much more complicated than that. In our culture, how we look affects our sense of self and our ability to take action in a very powerful way."

In survey settings, people rated those with attractive bodies as having a 59 percent greater chance of having a good marriage and a 48 percent greater chance of having a successful career than those with less attractive bodies. (Bush et al. 2001)

Remember, Ginkgo Biloba
Won't Help You Remember

Ginkgo biloba, extract from leaves of the ginkgo tree, is marketed world-wide as an enhancer of memory and other mental functions. A total of $500 million worth of ginkgo biloba is sold per year in the United States alone. There is, however, no science to back up the marketing claims.

YOU'RE IN A shopping center, and you've forgotten where you parked the car. You're on your way to work and you can't remember if you locked the door. You're watching a movie and you can't remember where you've seen the actor before.

"Don't worry. It's normal," says David Salmon, University of California, San Diego neuropsychologist. "Especially as we get older, our brains just work less efficiently. Things we could remember effortlessly when we were younger require more effort when we get older."

But it's not hopeless. "Once something is registered in the brain, an older person can retain it over time as well as a young person," Salmon says. "It's just that you need to focus more."

"Any kind of preoccupation or stress makes it difficult to pay attention and have deep memory encoding," says Larry Squire, a professor of psychiatry at the University of California, San Diego. "How well you pay attention at the time of learning information determines how well you will remember it."

"Don't look to ginkgo biloba and other supplements to enhance your memory," Dr. Salmon says. "Research has concluded they're a waste of money."

Using an experimental setup in which half the participants took ginkgo biloba and half took a placebo, researchers found that there were no measurable differences between the two groups' memory or mental functions. (Memory Clinic 2002)

Think About Potential

You do not have to solve every problem that comes up, and you should not strive for the complete absence of disagreements. But you must always keep part of your attention focused on hope, on the possibility that whatever difficulties arise today will be solved, forgotten, or at least less important in the future.

PATRICIA RECALLS RETURNING to her home from work one evening to find her husband, Eric, sitting in the dark alone. "My life is over," he said. "I have no real purpose anymore."

A month earlier, Eric had taken an early-retirement package and enthusiastically left his high-stress job. At the time, Patricia's own career was peaking. "I understood that Eric missed his professional environment, the prestige of being an authority in his field, and even the business travel he used to complain about so much," she says. "He used to get phone calls from all over the country asking for his advice with business problems," Patricia says. "Now I'm asking him what he's making for dinner.

"But I took his unhappiness as an insult. After all, he was married to me."

Eric found his stride a few months later. "I saw that I have fewer stresses and demands than ever. Any stress I have, it's because I choose to have it," he says. "There's a great deal of happiness if you look for it. I can see that now. That was the life we led and enjoyed then; this is the one we enjoy now."

A strong belief in relationship efficacy—that the relationship can continue to move forward and meet both partners' goals—is an aspect of nearly nine in ten relationships that continue successfully into long-term commitments. (Thomas 1999)

You'll Get What You're Afraid Of

When we spend time worrying about things that could go wrong, we're not spending time trying to improve. Which means, worrying about things going wrong increases the chances that they will go wrong. Accepting that sometimes we will succeed and sometimes fail frees us to pursue achievements and to spend time thinking about what we can do instead of what we can't.

"MOST BUSINESS IS built on a foundation of rejection. If a business hired everyone who applied for its jobs, or bought every product a salesman offered it, then it would be bankrupt in ten minutes," says Martin, an acting coach who has counseled hundreds of budding thespians. "Unless you don't want anything, you'll have to learn how to love rejection, because it will be coming.

"There isn't an actor you've heard of, there isn't an actor alive, who hasn't been rejected for more parts than they'll ever get.

"It doesn't mean that you love to lose," Martin believes, "but that you embrace the process that gets you to the outcome you want. And rejection is just a step in the process."

Employees who spent "a lot" of time worrying about their job were 17 percent less productive than workers who "seldom" or "never" worried about their job. (Verbeke and Bagozzi 2000)

See the Beauty Around You

It could be a flower. It could be a work of art. It could be the greatest pass you've ever seen a quarterback throw. Take time to truly see the things that inspire you. Take time to fit them into your life every day. There is beauty, however you define it, in the world around you.

DAVID SAW THE roses he gave his wife on their anniversary from a whole different vantage point than most people.

Looking at them in a vase, the amateur photographer wondered what kind of picture he might be able to create if he took an extreme close-up of a single perfect petal. He positioned his camera only inches away from the flower, and created a photo in which one petal fills the entire frame.

When he saw the developed photo, he was excited with what he had. "The close-up has the effect of distorting what you are looking at," David says. "If you didn't know it was a rose petal, you wouldn't immediately recognize what this was a photo of. When it becomes abstract like that, I think it reveals a different kind of beauty than what you had with the entire flower."

David dedicates most of his photographic efforts to nature scenes. Nature photography, he thinks, is a more creative process, one that requires him to really stop and soak in his environment and hone in on the beauty in it.

"And, unlike when you photograph people, seldom do trees complain that you didn't get them from a flattering angle," David says.

Those who said they regularly took notice of something beautiful were 12 percent more likely to say they were satisfied with their lives. (Isaacowitz, Vaillant, and Seligman 2003).

Whet Your Appetite for Success

If you spend your time worrying and impatiently awaiting an easy life, or attempt to pursue something you don't really care about, you will reduce your appetite for success. Cultivate your instincts in the direction you want them to lead you, and your growing motivation will make the pursuit of success easier to live with.

"I WAS THE kind of student that really upset a teacher," says Herbert Brennan, "because they believed I could be a good student, but I never tried very hard.

"All through high school, I was no more than mediocre—listlessly going through the motions of chemistry, algebra, history, English, and the rest.

"I was barely admitted to the local state college, and when I got there, I loafed my way through the placement exams, barely scoring outside of the remedial range."

Sometime early in his freshman year, Herbert says, everything changed: "I remember the feeling to this day because it was so shocking. I was sitting down to read a book for my history class, and it hit me that I was happy about it. I was looking forward to opening the book and investing myself in it."

Herbert went from there to graduating with honors with a degree in history, and then onto graduate school, ultimately to become a professor. "I became a different student when I found a subject I loved, and I was unstoppable once I knew what it was," he says.

Long-term studies of motivation find that people are capable of reducing or improving their level of motivation by as much as 58 percent during their careers. (Alderman 1999)

Write Through Pain

Illness can be more than we can handle. One way to help yourself process what's happening to you without becoming overwhelmed is to write down your thoughts in a personal journal. Writing about our lives helps reduce our stress level and can actually improve our overall health.

KIRK TEACHES PEOPLE how to record their thoughts, their feelings, their daily events, or whatever else might be on their mind in a journal. Kirk doesn't work for a school or college; he works for a hospital.

"Writing about illness and traumatic events helps patients to finally deal with and accept what has happened, and that process reduces stress and sleeplessness," Kirk say. "By altering the physiological stress patterns in their bodies, their health improves.

"People need to have a place for their personal voice. Writing allows you to find answers to daunting problems within yourself, rather than having to rely on answers from others. Through that, you get a sense of empowerment."

Whatever type of journal, the rules are the same: there are none. "We all suffer from English major's disease," Kirk says. "Forget about outlines, grammar, even punctuation. The journal is not about school or grades. It's all for you."

Kirk recommends getting started by setting a timer and writing for at least eight minutes about whatever comes to mind. And you don't have to look at your journal as a daily obligation. "A journal is the kind of friend you want it to be: an every-day phone call or occasional get-together," Kirk says.

A research project asked people suffering from chronic conditions such as asthma and arthritis to write about their lives in a journal for an hour per week. Forty-seven percent of the patients had a clinically relevant improvement in symptoms in the months after they started their journals. (North Dakota State University 1999)

To Find a Better Way, Look Where You've Been

Sigmund Freud argued a century ago that, good or bad, the model for our human interactions was cast in the experiences of youth and was likely to be repeated throughout our lives. Unless you make an effort to think about what you are doing and why, you are likely to repeat yourself, often to the detriment of your relationships.

WHEN FORMER SPEAKER of the House Newt Gingrich told his second wife he had been seeing another woman and wanted a divorce, he didn't mention that the affair he'd started had been going on for six years. "I found out with the rest of the country watching a news conference held by his lawyers," says Marianne Gingrich.

Marianne was shocked. It was hard to speak of the end of her eighteen-year marriage and her husband's affair. "I don't have any way to express it," she says.

During the divorce proceedings, she found out that the affair began when she was frequently out of state caring for her terminally ill mother.

"Marianne thought that they had a very sound marriage, right up until this unexpected demand for divorce," her attorney says. He notes that Newt Gingrich served his first wife with divorce papers while she was in the hospital recovering from cancer surgery. "Mr. Gingrich has a very disposable view of loved ones. When they no longer serve his purposes, he trades them in. From what I understand, this has been his practice all his adult life," he adds.

People who say they had strong feelings of personal security in youthful relationships are 31 percent more likely to be socially supportive in their adult relationships than are people who did not feel personally secure as a child. (Lawrence 2001)

Tell Clean Jokes

Humor captures people's attention and sets them at ease. There is a major difference between positive humor and negative humor, however. Negative humor involves attacks on people or their ideas or areas of behavior that would not be discussed at the dinner table. Positive humor involves silliness, and if there is any target of the humor at all, it is the joke teller. In the workplace, use positive humor freely and negative humor not at all.

LOUIS SIEGFRIED RUNS a multimillion-dollar mail-order business selling computers. While he takes his business very seriously, he also takes having a positive attitude very seriously.

"I think if you have fun, then you do well. We can't tolerate people who aren't enthusiastic," Louis says.

Louis seeks employees who want to work, and a workplace where they'll want to work.

"Whether it's meetings, memos, or policies, most business seems to operate on the premise that if you can possibly make something boring, make it extra-boring. We operate under the rule that the best way to get people to do their job well is to get them to want to do their job, and the best way to do that is to make sure there's a little fun in what we do," Louis says.

When negative humor is used in the workplace, it tends to spread throughout the organization. Forty-one percent see it as a source of division in their office. Widespread positive humor, on the other hand, increases job satisfaction by 5 percent. (Decker and Rotondo 1999)

Turn Off the TV

Watching television is a very passive activity for our bodies and our brains. Unlike just about anything else we might choose to do with our time, viewing television requires almost no thought or action. It has the equivalent effect on our brains that sitting on the couch has on our bodies. Turn off the television, especially when there isn't something you specifically want to watch, and go do something, anything, else. It will make you healthier.

FLOUNDERING WHILE SHE waits for her job prospects to improve, Jody spends at least ten hours every day watching TV. The shows are generally the same: talk shows until noon, then news, then as many *Law & Order* reruns as she can find. Most weekends, channel-surfing is all the exercise Jody gets.

Jody knows her fascination with television is in many ways dangerous. She knows she can't allow the TV to become her only window on the outside world. But by the time she dies, Jody estimates, she will have spent at least a quarter of her life sitting in front of the tube.

Her situation seems to become increasingly frustrating to her. "I just want other people to know. Don't just sit around on the sofa thinking one day everything is going to be OK. That's how I let my life slip by, and now I regret it," Jody says.

Jody flips through some old photos of herself, contemplating all the time she has spent wasting away in her bedroom watching TV. "I will never get any of that time back," she says. "I could have done so much. I really would have liked to have had more of a life."

Excessive television viewing in middle age triples the danger of developing brain diseases such as Alzheimer's later in life. (Case Western Reserve University 2002)

Don't Bring Your Job Home with You

Working as hard as you possibly can is not working as well as you possibly can. When the workday is over, the work must recede from your thoughts and time.

JAMES KELLER DESIGNS home offices—spaces in existing rooms, or entire rooms dedicated to working from home. He thinks the home-office concept is a metaphor for the home/office worker.

"The space I design has to serve two functions. It has to be a home part of the day and an office part of the day," James says. "When you think about it, that is just what the person is, too: a family member part of the day and a worker part of the day.

"This is a limitation in a sense, since the design has to incorporate both functions. But it is also a strength, because, done right, it serves the greater need."

James says his emphasis is on making the space something that really exceeds people's needs, not just minimally functions: "I don't want to make a design that people can suffer through. I want to make something people can enjoy, someplace you want to be."

James's concept of a home office is not a space that beacons you to the office at all hours of the day. "You have to turn off the office lights and shut the door, and then see your house as a home come five o'clock. You might say, 'I work in that room from nine to five. Come five o'clock, I'll clean up, and it becomes a family room again,'" James says.

Workaholics—people who never seem to stop working or thinking about work—are three times more likely to say that their personal lives are unsatisfying. (Porter 2001)

Practice Maintenance for Life

We don't buy a house or a car and expect it to stay in good working order over the years without regular upkeep and repairs. Yet we often think our relationships will keep going regardless of how we treat them. Give your relationships, whether with friends or family, regular attention and effort so that what you value will keep on being there for you.

"EVERYBODY I KNOW has a good friend, someone they were very close to, and then lost touch with. I was committed to trying to avoid that with these guys," says Tony, by way of explanation for the twenty-second annual edition of the *Seventh Avenue News.*

As boys, Tony says, he and his buddies grew up together in Brooklyn: "We all had plans. We were going to do this, see that, takeover this."

School, jobs, and the military quickly scattered the group. But Tony paid careful attention to his friends' addresses, and would write them from time to time. "Soon the letters back and forth were filled with questions like, 'Have you heard from Mickey, what's he up to?' I decided that, rather than sharing the scattered information with each other one at a time, it made more sense to write it all down once," Tony says.

Thus was born the *Seventh Avenue News*—filled with the goings-on of the buddies, their lives, their families, and their friendships.

Mickey says he's grateful for Tony's efforts: "Because of Tony, the people I considered friends for life when I was a boy really are friends for life. They have been a part of the major events of my life."

People who said that maintaining the health of their relationships was a priority were 22 percent more likely to find their social lives satisfying. (Weigel and Ballard-Reisch 1999)

Don't Pack Like a Mule

Travelers often load themselves down with heavy baggage and plow ahead with little concern about how their habits affect their bodies. People were not meant to move vast quantities of luggage, especially slung over the shoulder.

"SHOULDERS TAKE MORE wear and tear today than ever before. Toting travel bags, luggage, laptop computers, backpacks, sports equipment, and musical instruments places stress on the shoulders that can lead to muscle strain and lower-back pain," explains Dr. Vernon Tolo, president of the American Academy of Orthopaedic Surgeons.

The American Academy of Orthopaedic Surgeons has found that four out of five adults experience lower-back pain and that problems in the lower back are the most frequent cause of lost workdays in adults under the age of forty-five.

"The best treatment for shoulder stress and strain is prevention," Dr. Tolo says. "Increasing muscle strength in your shoulders and daily stretching are essential, but selecting the right shoulder packs and using them properly are equally important. The right pack lightens the load and reduces the stress." Dr. Tolo recommends that people take advantage of luggage with wheels and of bags made out of lightweight material. "But if you must carry," he adds, "make sure you walk in an upright position and don't allow the bag to pull you to one side."

You should not carry more than 15 percent of your body weight on your shoulders and back. (American Academy of Orthopaedic Surgeons 2002)

Look for Value

People present themselves to us, and our natural inclination is to size them up—to create some kind of immediate impression of their personal abilities and liabilities. More important, we hold on to these often vague and hasty conclusions, and utilize them later. This means we can mistakenly overlook the talents of people we have already written off based on superficial information.

YEARS WENT BY, and Jane wondered if anybody was ever going to ask her to do anything more challenging than count. Her job was to monitor the assembly lines at a cosmetics manufacturer. Each hour she took note of the production level of each line, then sent the information to the floor manager.

Jane counted output, matched it with a count of materials used, and then did it all over again. Nobody asked her why the lines were slow or fast. That wasn't her job. Just count.

Over the course of five years, Jane took note of a hundred factors that influenced the pace of the lines. Factors she knew nobody else was paying attention to. For one, if the volume on the radio system was too low, the workers spoke to each other more often, slowing down their pace.

The general manager casually asked her one time how things were going, expecting a generic response. Instead, he nearly fell over when Jane said production was down 2 percent and offered a list of the three most likely explanations.

Jane was finally visible to management and was promoted to a job where she could put to use the observations she'd made over the years.

Sixty-one percent of successful business leaders say that one of their key characteristics is a willingness to engage in the revitalization of employees, actively attempting to see what workers are capable of and then helping them achieve that. (Boyer 1999)

Never Trade Your Morals for Your Goals

People who compromise what they believe in to satisfy their goals wind up dissatisfied with their accomplishments. If you do not believe yourself to be moral, satisfaction is unattainable.

TO MOST PEOPLE in the company, he was a distant memory or a historical figure looking down from his portrait on the wall. But Leonard Spacek, who ran the accounting firm Arthur Andersen from the 1940s through the 1970s, had always been clear on the importance of integrity to accounting. "The most serious problems in our profession are caused by our own self-indulgence," he had famously said.

Spacek was more than the leader of the firm; he became the leading voice of the industry. He said accounting firms must overcome the temptation to put selling additional services to a client ahead of providing their primary duty. He warned that putting a business decision ahead of an accounting decision would ultimately destroy both accounting and the business. His own company would prove him right.

Today, Arthur Andersen no longer exists. It lost the ability to continue as an accounting firm after it was prosecuted for helping Enron manipulate its profit statements, which came on the heels of several other accounting scandals in which Arthur Andersen allowed bogus financial statements to be issued by other companies.

"There is only one reason Arthur Andersen is gone," says one employee. "Greed."

People who consider themselves highly moral are 28 percent more likely to consider themselves happy than people who think their moral standards need to be improved. (Schminke, Ambrose, and Neubaum 2005)

Don't Let Irritation Be Louder Than Joy

Which is more important, good or bad? Regardless of your answer, bad is often a bigger part of our thoughts. The traffic jam that bogs down our day stays in our thoughts longer than the open road that sped us on our way. The rude clerk is memorable long after the nice clerk is forgotten. Remind yourself to see the good, to think about the good, to remember the good. Good is out there just as much as bad, but we are often prone to miss it.

KATHERINE TEACHES A course on stress reduction. She sees people burdened with frustrations and tensions that overwhelm them. "You can get to a point where there's almost nothing else in your life. And by that point, your entire system, mental and physical. will be jeopardized," Katherine says.

Katherine asks her students to talk about some of the stressful moments they faced that day. There's never a shortage of examples.

Katherine tells the class to think about all that they've heard from each other. "There is an infinite quantity of stress available to us if we choose to pursue it. The good news is we don't have to take all this stress on," Katherine says.

Katherine offers practical tips for her students to avoid compounding the worst moments of their day into their worst day: "First, take a deep breath. Deep breathing helps calm us down. Second, watch your thoughts. Negative or fearful thoughts create more anxiety and stress, and when you start heading down that road, change the subject for yourself. Third, give yourself an alternative. Practice visualization, and think about what you like and what you want to happen."

Among those over fifty, the hassles of the day were three times more prominent in their thinking than the pleasant moments of the day. (Hart 1999)

Sleep Well

Sleep is fuel for our systems that we were not made to do without. As is the case with food and water, we cannot simply skimp for a day and make up for it the next. Our bodies expect a steady supply of sleep and function best when provided with a full night's sleep every day.

MILITARY LEADERS HAVE identified a long-ignored but very important threat to soldiers: lack of sleep. Lt. Col. Jim Chartier of the U.S. Marines called sleep deprivation "our biggest enemy. It makes easy tasks difficult."

Brain scans show that a missed night of sleep will cause a metabolic drop in the prefrontal cortex—the section of the brain responsible for higher-order reasoning and judgment. For soldiers and pilots, that means that the part of the brain that discerns friend from foe, chooses targets, and navigates through a battlefield is truly addled by sleep loss.

Col. Gregory Belenky of the U.S. Army warns, "With little sleep, troops can doze off during chemical attacks, while on watch, or while operating dangerous equipment—and in wartime, it is all dangerous equipment."

Col. Belenky's research found that a single night without sleep can render a subject slow to react, easy to distract, and very forgetful. "The sleepless subject becomes impulsive, irritable, and unable to respond to complex problems with any but the most rote of responses," he says. Even more alarming, he adds, "without sleep, people have no grasp on the extent of their impairment."

Forty percent of adults are so sleepy during the day that it interferes with their daily activities. The National Sleep Foundation reports that sleep deprivation triggers a 10 to 35 percent drop in antibodies and immune cells. Sleep is essential for the repair of immune cells. People should aim for at least eight hours of sleep a night, more if they are sick. (National Sleep Foundation 2003)

Recognize the Value of Shared Values

Your core values were formed a long time ago and will likely be yours for the rest of your life. The same is true for the other person in a relationship. Given that neither of you is likely to change your core beliefs, it helps if those beliefs are compatible. Strong relationships depend on trust and communication. When you have similar beliefs, it feels safer and more rewarding to share your thoughts and feelings.

AS HER HUSBAND puts it, "Some people enter a room and the entire area seems to light up. Jane is definitely one of those people. She is vibrantly alive."

When Jane Douglass White was thirty, she had successful living in the palm of her hand. She was happily married, the mother of two healthy children, an accomplished songwriter, and the associate producer of the network TV show *Name That Tune.*

"The sky's the limit," she thought at the time.

Then the words of the physician changed everything: "You have cancer and must have surgery immediately." It felt like a death sentence, because Jane didn't know anyone who had recovered from cancer.

Although he was wracked with fears, her husband offered her comfort and strength throughout the long ordeal of treatment. To Jane, her recovery is nothing short of a miracle, a miracle she could never have endured without the steadying hand of her husband.

"He saw what was most important. That we both lived in love, instead of hate; in forgiveness, instead of resentment. And that no illness could change the fundamental bond of our lives together," Jane says.

The degree to which couples have similar values does not change over the course of their relationship. Those with similar values, however, are 22 percent more likely to rate their communication habits positively. (Acitelli, Kenny, and Weiner 2001)

Get Your Motivation Where You Can Find It

People who care do a better job in everything they do. Some people are driven internally by their own competitive juices. Some are driven externally by their thirst for approval and appreciation. Some are driven by a desire to succeed for their families. Some are driven by a desire to succeed to show up their families. Use what you really care about to make yourself passionate about how things turn out.

"I'D RATHER BECOME a furniture mover" is how seventy-year-old Lorna responded when her doctor told her she needed to exercise regularly. She said exercise would bore her out of her mind.

Lorna and her doctors realized that exercising was so unappealing to Lorna that she was unlikely to follow through with it on her own.

Her doctors helped place her in a women's exercise group that met three times a week at the University of Wisconsin.

While she was no great fan of the exercise regimen, it was the fifty other women in the group who first changed Lorna's attitude. "The wonderful women kept me coming back," she says. "It's one of the neatest groups of women I've ever met in my life. They have depth to them."

Over time, the rewards of the exercise brought their own joy to Lorna's life. "When I first started with this group I had back trouble and had laser surgery on my knee and a lot of pains and stiffness. But I'm back now. I can twirl and jitterbug every bit as good as I did when I was a kid. So that's amazing," Lorna says.

While level of motivation is highly correlated with success, the source of motivation varies greatly between individuals and is unrelated to success. (Bashaw and Grant 1994)

Have Some Tea with Your Remodeling

Remodeling efforts, including any painting or gluing, generally result in an unhealthy buildup of chemicals in the home. Dry tea bags will absorb chemicals in the air and reduce the amount of time it takes for a home to return to having healthy air quality.

SERENA FELL IN love with a very old house in central Philadelphia. It needed plenty of attention, Serena thought, but she could not resist it. Now she's making her way through it one room at a time—patching, painting, refinishing the hardwood floors, putting in new moldings and fixtures. "I love the old-style design of the house, but there's something to be said for walls without holes in them, and an update on fifty-year-old faded paint," she says.

Unfortunately for Serena, the fumes and smells produced by her efforts are hard to deal with: "It smells like I live in a factory or a refinery."

While she leaves the windows open as much as possible, that is not the most attractive solution during Philadelphia winters. "You can either air out the place and freeze, or keep the place warm while you choke on the air," Serena says.

Then Serena read about the tea-bag solution: "Tea bags are porous and soak up what's around them. Now I spread tea bags throughout the room I'm working in. Much of the stink goes right into the bags. I would say it cuts in half the time it takes for a room to stop smelling of paint and varnish."

The only challenge for Serena is putting up with the strange look she gets at the supermarket when she buys twenty boxes of tea.

Researchers found that scattering tea bags throughout a newly remodeled room reduced the toxicity level of chemicals in the air by up to 90 percent. (Tokyo Metropolitan Consumer Center 2002)

We Assume Similar Preferences

It's difficult to figure out what other people are thinking and feeling. As a shortcut for doing just that, we look to our own thoughts and feelings, and assume that the other person's are pretty close to our own. But our feelings are not representative of everyone else's—or of anyone else's, for that matter. When we project our feelings onto someone else, we wind up offering our response to our feelings.

JOYCE AND RICK did not see eye to eye when their teenage son stayed out past his curfew. "Every time this happened, we would wind up in a major disagreement about how to respond," says Joyce.

They disagreed not only on how to respond with regard to punishment, but even on the tone of their comments. From Joyce's vantage point, when Rick "sits down with our son, it's like they're discussing movies and sports instead of unacceptable behavior." But from Rick's position, Joyce makes "every mistake into a disaster."

Finally it became clear to both that the source of their problem was how differently they understood the situation. Rick took it as a good sign that their son didn't try to sneak in when he broke curfew, that his honesty was ultimately more important than the rules. Joyce was alarmed that if a small rule like a curfew was meaningless now, bigger rules would fall later. Talking through this, they realized that they came up with different answers to the situation because they saw a different situation. "We're still not completely on the same page, but we are far less baffled by each other's reaction now," Joyce says.

Across both relationships and friendships, more than eight in ten people assume a similarity of reaction between themselves and others in rating everyday things they liked and disliked. (Watson, Hubbard, and Wiese 2000b)

Memories Are Not Lost

Why do we forget something just when we want to remember it most? Why do we remember it hours or days later, when we had stopped trying to remember? Memories exist within your brain; they are not lost. However, we sometimes have trouble accessing those memories. Our brain is organized to store information in small pieces. The process can be interrupted by, among other things, our anxiety to remember. Trust yourself; the information is in there and it will come out. You may sometimes just have to wait.

GEORGE IS GREAT with names. He remembers them by breaking down new information into familiar images. An ardent sports enthusiast, he remembers that Gutzon Borglum designed Mount Rushmore, for example, by thinking of tennis champ Bjorn Borg and major league baseball player Mike Lum. "Whenever I think of Mount Rushmore, in my mind I automatically see Borg with his scraggly little beard and Mike Lum," he says.

For Sally, it often helps to associate the name with a physical feature or a trigger word. If it rhymes, all the better. Barry with the thick, wavy hair, can be remembered as Hairy Barry.

Dr. Harold Wolf of the University of Utah explains that an inability to remember something is just like coming upon a road closure and having to look for alternative routes. "If a stored memory is blocked for some reason, the brain will look for different connections in order to retrieve that information. Memory techniques are simply mental detours to get to where you want to go," says Dr. Wolf.

By measuring the electrical rhythms that parts of the brain use to communicate with each other, researchers have demonstrated that our memory of a single object requires our brain to access multiple bits of information. Therefore, the inability to remember something is not forgetting; it is an obstacle between the different pieces of information. (University of Arkansas 2002)

Nobody Wins Without a Loser

On the path to success, you will sometimes confront situations in which you must directly compete with someone, and your victory over them will create bitterness. Even more frequently, your success will cause others to compare themselves to you and to react with jealousy at your ability. Take comfort in the knowledge that this is not a personal attack on you, but instead a sincere but unpleasant form of flattery.

"EVERY YEAR, I spend less time talking around the water cooler," says Sheila. "As you advance up the corporate ladder, a lot of people begin to think of you as the enemy, instead of a friend who happens to have been promoted."

Sheila struggles with the implications of her rapid rise through the ranks of the financial-services company where she works.

"At the same time, you can't sit around wishing away success so that your co-workers would like you again," she says.

The best advice on the matter came from her father, who toiled for forty-five years without achieving the advancements his daughter had in less than ten. He said to Sheila, "Treat everyone with respect, and don't treat anyone, above or below you, based on their station. Eventually, that respect will come back to you."

Six in ten top managers report that they have lost friendships among co-workers who were not promoted as fast as they were. (Austin 2000)

If You're Not Sure, Guess Positively

Unhappy people take a situation in which they are not sure and come to a negative conclusion. If they aren't certain if another person is being nice, they assume the person must have a hidden, selfish agenda. Happy people take that same situation and guess the positive possibility—that is, that the person really is nice.

HENRY IS A seventy-two-year-old man who always had a good word for his neighbors. He lived modestly in southwestern Arkansas in a small home with only a woodstove for heat. Over the years, Henry watched his home deteriorate steadily. But he had too little energy and too little money to make repairs.

One of his neighbors organized a group to virtually rebuild Henry's house, giving it modern heat and improving the plumbing. Henry was stunned by their efforts. Why were all these people taking such an interest in his house? What did they have to gain?

Any situation can be viewed as an act of selfishness if we try hard enough. But doing so would make us cold, critical, and cynical. And there's no way out of it, because a person we view negatively cannot do anything to improve our impression of them. We need to consider that our perspective on what motivates people can be either a source of comfort to us or a source of alarm.

Henry's ultimate conclusion is clear. "These were just good people doing a good thing, and I thank them for it," Henry says.

When an unhappy person must interpret the world, eight in ten times he or she will see the negative in an event. When a happy person must interpret the world, eight in ten times he or she will see the positive. (Brebner 1995)

Understand What You're Looking For

People have basic ideas about the world and their place in it. To better understand what you need from a relationship, think about who you are. Your interests, your beliefs, your career choice—all are indicators of your fundamental personality. Remember, your choices about things other than relationships reveal a lot about what you need from a relationship.

IN 1953, JAMES Watson helped discover the structure of DNA, the building block of life. He had youth, fame, and a brilliant future. What didn't he have? A girlfriend.

A whiz in the lab, he was a mess at romance. "I was immature," Watson says. Outside the lab, he was just another lonely guy hoping to connect. "I was like everyone else," he adds.

"This is what a scientist's life is like," says Watson. "It's not just great ideas or great moments." On the contrary, he says, scientists—including him—hatch "a lot of failed ideas" and too often chase "enthusiasms of the last twenty-four hours that aren't worth the effort."

Women, however, still were a mystery. "This was true even though men are somehow programmed to think about women about 90 percent of the time," he declares.

It took years of searching, but James Watson finally met his future wife, Elizabeth Lewis, a "beautiful girl with a passion for science." She understood his passion for ideas and shared his enthusiasms for new ideas. Elizabeth was also willing to overlook what he considers to be one of his defining talents: "I know how to irritate people, boy."

People's occupational direction was among the best predictors of their views on relationship roles, with those in nurturing professions being 47 percent more likely to take a nurturing view of their relationship role. (Klute et al. 2002)

See Your Goals

Goals give us focus and purpose. Regardless of what is important to you now, your goals should be clear and visible every day.

IN MORE THAN three decades as a newspaper photographer, Bob Jordan has photographed hurricanes, governors, presidents, a war, and championship basketball games. Bob says that the key to his career has been a constant dedication to the goal of doing his job as well as he can. Bob took seriously his father's belief that nothing in work is guaranteed, but that "the one thing you can control is how hard you work.'"

Today Bob is recognized as a mentor to countless photojournalists. And even with all the experience he has, he still gets to events before his colleagues in the media arrive so that he is better prepared and set on his plan for getting the right shot. And even though he's a skilled veteran in the trade, "I'm nervous before every assignment," Bob says. "I've never lost that, whether it's going out and shooting a head shot or covering a basketball game. Your name goes on the picture. I want it to be the best it can be.

"Some people might try to coast as they get older. But that's not for me. I don't see why, as you get older, you can't get better."

People who can identify a goal they are currently pursuing are 19 percent more likely to feel satisfied with their lives and 26 percent more likely to feel positive about themselves. (Krueger 1998)

Short-Term Stress Is Healthy

Our bodies are meant to deal with short-term stress. For short-term stress, adrenaline surges within us, and our immune system is heightened. A short-term stress, such as having to give a speech, has a defined ending point such that the adrenaline surge can stop and the body can return to normal.

THE SEASON FOR a professional football player is only sixteen games long. While each game lasts about three hours, the actual time spent on the field with the ball in play amounts to no more than about six minutes per game. That means a star player's season is based on success in just over an hour and a half of effort spaced out over several months. An entire career can take as little as ten hours of actual in-game action.

Of course there are countless hours of practice and conditioning before those games take place, but the measure of an athlete will be performance in those games. How does an athlete deal with the incredible weight of having to provide an outstanding performance in such a limited time frame.

"That is really the positive side of stress," says psychologist Gary Foley. "We are all capable of doing more than we imagine in short bursts.

"The key, though, is that they are short bursts. If you asked a football player to play a game seven days a week, he would collapse before the week was out," Dr. Foley says.

"Short bursts of effort are healthy stressors. They focus us. They are not just productive; they are healthy. It's good for the circulation system. Good for the immune system. And it's good for just a little bit at a time," Dr. Foley adds.

Researchers found that short-term stress boosts the body's ability to fight disease. However, prolonged stress weakens the immune system by as much as 60 percent. (University of Michigan 2002b)

Prepare for Milestones

Milestone events—births, deaths, career changes, children leaving home—inspire reflection. These events encourage us to look at ourselves and our relationships, and they often lead us to question the path we have taken. This experience is jolting, however, because it is unexpected. Reduce the significance of these occasions by reflecting regularly, regardless of whether a milestone event is at hand.

NEW YORKERS CAROL and Bill were, in their own words, coasting through marriage together. When their two sons moved out of the family home within weeks of each other, both Carol and Bill fell into a deep contemplation of their journey together.

"We both realized we were getting worn out," says Bill. "We kept running into the same arguments and roadblocks. It was getting tiresome."

Carol adds, "We had kind of fallen into mediocrity, like, 'Ho-hum, this is it for married people.' The passion, the electricity, the vibrance of being in love was in the past."

To heal the distance they both felt between them, they decided to take twenty minutes every day to do nothing but share their feelings—about everything, from the world to each other. And, Carol says, they write each other notes: "When you are just getting started, there's always a nice or sometimes inspiring note being written. Twenty years later the only note you'll get says 'Buy milk at the market.' We decided to change that.

"I vowed my life to Bill forever, that he should be my number one priority," says Carol. "When you put everything into perspective, twenty minutes a day is not that radical to improve your life."

People are eight times more likely to question the health of their relationship in the aftermath of a major life event than they are in general. (Schwartz 2000)

Your Health Isn't Just About You

O ur health is not just a reflection of our habits; it's also a reflection of our lifestyle and the people around us. People who enjoy good, strong relationships are healthier because they feel less stress generally and tend to deal with stressful situations better. Cherishing your relationships with family and friends is as important to your health as eating right and exercising.

LEILA IS A nurse. She knows how to spot the danger signs that indicate someone's health is at risk, and she spends part of her workweek trying to educate people about the warning signs they should be looking for in their family, friends, and neighbors.

"People think in terms of having enough food and proper shelter. We think we can immediately recognize problems. But no one sees loneliness. It doesn't happen when we are there checking in; it happens when we're not looking," Leila says.

Leila explains that loneliness is a condition with tremendous implications, not just for how we feel about ourselves, but for how we treat ourselves. "A lonely person is more likely to skip meals or eat less-healthy foods. A lonely person is more likely to avoid getting medical care when they are sick, and to ignore or forget to take medication. A lonely person is just willing to accept a lower standard of life for themselves," she says.

"Whether you are concerned about a lonely person or are a lonely person yourself," Leila says, "the best thing you can do is show someone you care. As soon as you crack that isolation that comes from feeling left out, feeling that no one cares, you begin to see people treating themselves better. Loneliness is a feeling, but it can be replaced by a better feeling."

Loneliness in otherwise healthy people was associated with increased blood pressure and decreased heart capacity. (University of Chicago 2002)

Don't Want Everything

Success in life is not a matter of getting everything, because that is impossible and wouldn't be much of a joy even if it were possible. Success is a matter of getting what you need.

Think of success as filling a box. You'll be finished sooner not just by working harder to fill it, but also by choosing a smaller box.

BECKY CONSIDERS HERSELF normal in most respects.

She has a career, a husband, two children, and almost no time.

"Do you ever feel like you woke up in an episode of *The Twilight Zone*? My story is the person who constantly has more things to do and less time in which to do them. It's like every day I have to make more runs to the store than the day before, and I have to do it in half the time," Becky says.

Becky concluded that the challenge to living life at her own pace instead of constantly in a rushed hurry was to "realize what is really important. I spent so much time doing things because I thought I was supposed to instead of because it was really necessary."

To get out of her own private Twilight Zone, Becky stopped going after everything. "If you run out of time trying to do absolutely everything, then sometimes you wind up finishing the stupid stuff and missing out on what really matters," she says.

What success means is not universal. Studies of people who have attained nearly identical achievements in the workplace, for example, find great variation in their levels of satisfaction, with some considering themselves tremendously successful and others considering themselves average, or even failures. (Maasen and Landsheer 2000)

Rest Up—This Is Going to Take Some Effort

All the behaviors that foster a strong relationship require not only effort but an ability to see things from your partner's perspective. All this effort is far harder, and far less likely to take place, when you are exhausted. Realize that rest is a required ingredient for you and your partner to find your time together satisfying.

KEITH GULPS COFFEE all night long. "Sweatshop is a good description," the veteran long-haul truck driver, husband, and father of four says in describing his job. "But I've got to do it. I'll probably kill myself putting my kids through college. But there's no way I'm ever going to let them drive a truck.

"We drive hard, putting in long hours day and night. We get paid by the mile, not by the hour. We get paid for delivery, really, not for what's necessary in between."

Truck drivers spend weeks away from home and family, living out of duffel bags and sleeping in the back of their rigs. "I know guys who are running so hard that they haven't been home in two months. Some are on their third and fourth marriages," Keith says.

"My wife wants me home for the weekend, but the company's got me headed in the opposite direction," he adds. "When I get there, I'll be so tired I wouldn't notice it if the couch were on fire. I'll sleep for a couple days, then head out for my next run. And my wife will say I wasn't ever really here."

Having driven 130,000 miles a year for many years, Keith has come to one conclusion: "Something's got to change."

People feeling excessively tired found that they were more likely to experience conflict in their relationships, and 25 percent were more likely to feel emotionally out of control. (Roberts and Levenson 2001)

Your Lives Must Fit Together

Ninety-nine percent of the parts of your car could be in perfect shape, but if the 1 percent includes a flat tire or a dead battery, your car can't be used. Much of your life can be healthy and satisfying, but if an important part of it is not, you will not feel fulfilled. Successful living is not a matter of success in the workplace or success at home; it is the product of their combination.

EDWIN AND VICKIE Weatherspoon began as partners in life and then became partners in business.

The California couple were married for three years when they decided Vickie should join her husband's business, which offers janitorial services for corporate clients.

Husband and wife working together—a dream come true? Hardly. "It was difficult at first," Vickie explains, since both had their ideas about how things should be done. "We're both power players. We'd step over boundaries and take it home."

They committed themselves over time to putting their two worlds in balance. "We learned to keep our personal lives separate and how to stay friends at the end of the day. By the same token, if we're at home or on vacation or out with friends, we won't be talking business all the time," Vickie says.

"The key to our success is the foundation we had first, that helps us keep perspective on what's really most important," she adds.

You might think that the best work year would be the worst home year. Instead, people at the peak of their careers report that reaching their goals in work increases their commitment to their home lives because they feel a great sense of security that improves their time outside of work. (Persley 1998)

Find a Physician You Like

It may sound superficial, but one of the most important things we need in a doctor is a quality we respond positively to. We need to have a good feeling about our doctors. For all their training and ability, if we feel disconnected from them, if we feel they think of us as a just another widget, we are less likely to seek their help and listen to their advice.

DON WAS HAVING trouble getting through to his doctor. He called several times and left messages, then didn't hear back. He debated whether he should start looking for a new doctor, but he also wondered whether perhaps he was overreacting.

When Don finally received an appointment, he arrived to find that his doctor was overbooked. After waiting all morning, Don finally saw his doctor for less than ten minutes.

So Don decided to do a little research. He was shocked to find out the doctors' own association, the American Medical Association, reported that as many as a quarter of patients switch doctors because of problems communicating with their doctors.

"I began to understand this wasn't just me," Don says. "Whether it seems no one is listening when you have an appointment or you can't get through to make an appointment, you feel like you don't matter when you can't communicate with your doctor."

Don says he found that the doctors' association offered various helpful hints for physicians in dealing with the personal side of the job: "The AMA says that the personal side, how they treat people, is where trust comes from. Without that trust, all the scientific knowledge in the world doesn't do the patient much good."

People who rated their physician friendly were two times more likely to seek medical attention at the first sign of distress and were three times more likely to follow medical instructions. (Auerbach, Penberthy, and Kiesler 2004)

Don't Let Secrets Eat You Up

While honesty might be thought of as the best policy, there are truths that might be too devastating to admit in a relationship. In situations in which you fear that the effects of the truth in your relationship might be devastating, seek a trusted confidant with whom you can discuss the truth and relieve your burden.

CORRINNA AND MANUEL were separated. If she told the right story, he'd never really need to know. She says she didn't even know what she was doing when she was caught.

Corrinna had become mixed up with the wrong people, and when she delivered a package for one of them, it led to an arrest and a six-month jail sentence. With her marriage in tatters already, she thought surely this would be the final straw. But she decided that the truth, and the shame of it, might do her some good. It was a hard thing for her to say out loud, but it was liberating. "The more I put it out there," she says, "the less power it has over me."

She dreamed of the moment she would be free and could return to her native Alaska. She imagined landing at the airport and being swept up in hugs upon arrival. After so much time "swallowing silent tears in dark places," as Corrinna calls it, she cried when she saw Manuel waiting for her.

An aspiring poet, Corrinna won a poetry competition just weeks after her release.

She persevered with a belief that she could overcome the cost of the truth, because, she says, "in a world so bleak, I needed idealism to stay on my feet."

Among people who have held important secrets from their partner, 27 percent report having had feelings of physical sickness from the discomfort of the deception. (Kelly and Carter 2001)

Remember the Difference Between You and Everybody Else

Your future is neither limited by the failures nor assured by the successes of those around you. Remember, *your* talents and *your* desires will create your future.

ANTHONY JOHNSON, A physics professor at the New Jersey Institute of Technology, works with lasers that travel at speeds measured in femtoseconds, which are a million times shorter than nanoseconds.

Until Anthony, the son of a bus driver, came of age, every male in the Johnson family drove a bus or a train for a living. Most everyone he knew growing up struggled just to keep up with the bills and keep a roof over their heads.

But Anthony saw a specific path for himself in high school, then college, and finally graduate school. And now he is on the lookout for the next generation of physicists.

"Too many young people have written science off; that's a real tough battle we have. But if we don't show students an example, they won't dream of careers in science or anything else. Too many give up, because there's so much give up around them.

"I wouldn't be here without some great people who invested in me and helped me see what I could do," Anthony explains. "And I'm not just going to sit here without going to the next generation and showing them what we do here. Because what we do could shape the future."

People who thought their future was likely to be very similar to that of their peers were 26 percent less likely to feel strongly optimistic about their careers. (Arnett 2000)

Be an Expert

Choose a particular area that is crucial to what you do, and learn everything you can about it. There is no better way to ensure that you will be invaluable and that your suggestions will be respected and followed.

FRED WILBER HAS sold quirky and hard-to-find music out of his store in Montpelier, Vermont, for twenty-seven years.

He worried that the Internet, and specifically the giant Web retailers who seemed to be able to sell everything, might spell the end of his business.

Instead, he decided to go online himself. Fred's has neither the resources nor the inclination to do battle with the Web superstores. Instead, his Web site is an online version of his physical store, featuring items that reflect his peculiar tastes and unmatchable knowledge of movie soundtracks.

And he's found that that's what's bringing in business. "You can go anywhere to buy the latest hit CD, but who is going to tell you about a great CD you've never heard of, and who is going to track down a copy of an out-of-print movie soundtrack of *Gordy! The Little Pig that Hit it Big!*? I can do those kinds of things that no one else can," Fred says.

By "focusing on our own niche, what we know best," Fred says, he has watched his combined in-store and online sales grow by over 10 percent a year, and his customer base by 20 percent.

Sixty-eight percent of people who consider themselves successful say that there is at least one area of their job in which they are an expert. (Austin 2000)

Root for the Home Team

Living with the ups and downs of your area's favorite sports team will help you feel a part of the community and show you how much you have in common with your neighbors.

BILL SAYS THERE is no rivalry in sports that matches Ohio State versus Michigan. When the two schools match up in football, the nation's sports fans are always excited—and nowhere more so than in Bill's hometown of Columbus. The people in Columbus, the home of Ohio State, are known to cover their homes and cars with Ohio State flags—and even to decorate their front yards with the school's Buckeye mascot.

"What's amazing is that it is something that almost everybody here has in common," Bill says. "You could be walking through the supermarket, hear three words of a conversation, and be able to join right in because it's about the game. If you left your house during the game, you'd hardly be able to find another person, because everyone's either watching it on TV or at the game."

Bill found himself with one source of discomfort about the big game, however. As luck would have it, he lives on probably the only street in town that seems out of place: Michigan Avenue. Bill contacted the city, and although they assured him the street was named for the state and not the school, they agree to temporarily rename it Buckeye Way during the month leading up to the game.

"Everybody on the block is excited—the street name fits us a lot better now," Bill says.

Rooting for a local sports team was found to have positive effects by providing a common interest with others in the community and increasing overall happiness by 4 percent. (Shank and Beasley 1998)

The Future Can Be Brighter Than the Past

In most things, we've taught ourselves to see tomorrow as an extension of today. Things that are true now will continue to be true. The sun will rise in the east. Autumn will follow summer. But we are not limited in our happiness by the patterns we set yesterday. Our happiness is the product not just of our life experiences, but of our perspectives on them. Yesterday is not the limit on our happiness today or tomorrow.

MAE SAW THE end of the nineteenth century, every day of the twentieth century, and then welcomed the twenty-first century.

Mae has long since outlived her many friends and nearly all of her family. But her perspective on that is clear: "Always look forward, never back.

"When I get up in the morning, it's a blessing to have been given the chance to see another day. And I think that it just might be a good one."

Mae thinks people, whether they are old enough to remember when Woodrow Wilson was president or are too young to remember life before cell phones, should focus on all the possibilities of today.

"Enjoy what you have today. Try to like the people around you and be good to them. Be kind, and lend a helping hand. Try new things. Most of all, enjoy yourself, and remember that it's always better to laugh than to cry," Mae says.

Two-thirds of those who characterized their experiences in childhood and young adulthood as unhappy reported that their lives in the fifties and beyond were happy. (Freeman, Templer, and Hill 1999)

Religion Can Help Ease Your Burden

Whether changing their lives to improve their health or dealing with their recovery from a health problem, people with strong religious beliefs benefit from the foundation of confidence and purpose that their beliefs provide.

"WE ALL WANT to be in control. But when you get to a V.A. hospital and you've got a foot wound that won't heal, you come to understand you're not in control," says Jon, an air force veteran.

Jon says his solution to seizing control in an uncontrollable situation is turning to his faith: "When you look to your faith, you have far more of a peace about life."

Dr. Harold Koenig of Duke University agrees: "Furious attempts to gain control over health conditions breed anxiety and depression. But religious beliefs provide an indirect form of control that helps interrupt the vicious cycle."

Dr. Koenig says the favorable impact religion has on health flows from the greater sense of purpose in life, a sense of control, social support, honorable living, and serenity. "The effects are completely explained by psychological, social, behavioral, and physiological mechanisms," he says.

"I think we're discovering that neither religion nor science is enough by itself," Dr. Koenig says. "You need to address the whole person. Not just their body. Not just their psychology. Not just their social or religious aspect. But all of these come together and influence each other, and you need to address the whole to get the best outcome."

A study found that people who make religion a significant part of their lives are 81 percent less likely to battle anxiety and depression and are more likely to have confidence that they can recover from an illness. (Columbia University 2003b)

Regrets Hold Us Back

We can't change the past; we can't improve it. Dwelling on past disappointments can change our future, but only to make it worse. Relieve yourself of the burden of past regrets. Your goal is to set the best course for the future, not to suffer over the imperfections of the past.

ON THE SURFACE, Nathan would be a good candidate for living with a heavy load of regret. He invested every penny he had, and then borrowed some more, to start a business that never prospered. He came home from work one day and found that his wife of twelve years had packed up her things and left. "Didn't even say good-bye," he recalls. Three years later, his home was flooded in a hurricane.

"You know what I regret?" Nathan asks. "Nothing.

"I don't pretend I didn't make mistakes. I made a lot. And it's clear I had some poor runs of luck. But the way I look at it, it's the good and the bad that made me who I am. If you go back and change something, who knows what you are left with?

"And thinking about what I've lost gets in the way of thinking about what I have, which is a long time in front of me to do things right, or do things better. I can't let regret stop me now. Then it would be all over for me."

Those who frequently thought about past mistakes and regrets were 17 percent less likely to feel happy with their lives. (Jokisaari 2003)

Your Teeth Are More Than Something to Chew On

We think of our teeth as existing in almost a separate medical world from the rest of our body. However, gum diseases can have consequences for the functioning of our entire body. In fact, our teeth and gums are a vitally important gateway to our coronary system. To take care of your body, you must take care of your teeth and gums. Brushing, flossing, and getting regular cleanings and checkups are key elements in the defense not only of our teeth but of our overall well-being.

DENTAL EXPERTS ARE looking beyond drilling, yanking teeth, and doing root canals to consider the importance of the mouth in assessing one's health. Specifically, they see evidence that identifying mouth microbes provides important clues to general health.

Researchers are learning to detect changes in the huge populations of bacteria, viruses, yeast cells, and other microbes that thrive in the mouth. "These bugs don't colonize your mouth in a random way," says Sigmund Socransky, a professor of periodontology at Harvard University. "Rather, they form in a pattern."

Professor Socransky noted it's a very good thing that certain microbes inhabit the mouth. The healthful bacteria tend to keep the harmful ones at bay, he says.

Professor Socransky's work has shown that shifts in microbe populations accompany disorders ranging from gum disease to heart disease, strokes, and pneumonia. The outcome of the efforts of bacteria-wielding toxins to annihilate competitors can influence dental health, he says. There are "good bugs that kill bad bugs. We'd love to replace the bad guys with good guys. But we don't know how to do that just yet."

People with periodontal disease are up to 57 percent more likely to suffer from heart problems. (University of Pittsburgh 2002)

Define What You Need

We don't start a relationship unless we have high expectations. How can a relationship built on such positive expectations turn into such a difficult struggle? For many of us, the traits that grab our attention, that make us think a relationship would be worth pursuing, are not the same things that will meet our needs and make us happy over time. Think about what you truly need from a relationship, and let that guide your relationship goals and decisions.

"THEY SAID IT was the opportunity of a lifetime," John remembers. "It was a promotion, a chance to run my own division, but it was also a transfer one thousand miles away."

John turned down the promotion to stay in his current position. "It was flattering, but it doesn't make sense right now," John says. Why? His wife, Liz, was immersed in the struggles of a first-year medical residency.

Liz works twelve-hour days and spends every fourth night on call at the hospital. The couple struggles to find a few hours of free time together. "It's kind of pathetic, but we have to get our schedules out, and I'll ask him what's a good day to take off," says Liz.

When she finally could take a week off, the couple went all the way to Africa for a safari vacation to escape the pressures of work.

But Liz was inspired by John's decision to defer his own career path. "It is really a testament to what's most important to him. He understands the big picture of our life together, and when my training is completed, I will move wherever he'd like to go," she says.

Researchers found that the traits that first attracted people to their partners were no longer relevant to 34 percent of them when they were asked again six months or more after they began dating. (Felmlee 2001)

You Can't Be Persistent Without Perspective

Most of the things you really want are not going to come to you overnight, this week, or next week. Most of what is truly important to you will take several years, sometimes a lot longer. How can you go on, knowing that you have so much farther to go on? Persistent people arm themselves with the knowledge that what they want can be done. They focus not on the distance they must go to get what they want but, instead, on the belief that what they want is possible.

SOMETIMES HE EVEN has trouble convincing his wife, but investment adviser John Conover tells everyone that the stock market is a great long-term investment.

"There is no better long-term investment. Disciplined, long-term investing in a diversified group of stocks is not sexy or thrilling—or likely to make you rich overnight. But then again, there isn't anything that's going to make you rich overnight," John says.

"Good companies with good products will make money, and in the long run their stock will appreciate. There will be dips, because of weak years for the company or the economy overall, but patience will guarantee that you hold the stock when the good years come. And the good years will outnumber the bad," he adds.

Trying for immediate returns out of stocks, however, is to John "a fool's game. It's hazardous to your financial health and is something I recommend only if you want to lose all your investments rather than make money."

In comparing people who tend to give up easily with people who tend to carry on, even through difficult challenges, researchers find that persistent people spend twice as much time thinking not about what has to be done but about what they have already accomplished, the fact that the task is doable, and that they are capable of it. (Sparrow 1998)

You'll Need Some Relationship Friends

You should try to form some relationship friends—other couples with some common interests who can interact as a couple with you and your partner. Relationship friends help ground us in the importance of our relationship and give us a fun and healthy outlet for activities built around other people but that include our partner.

BEFORE CHRIS GOT married to Susan, he regularly spent a lot of time with his single friends. "Before we got serious, I would have rather hung out with them," he says. "But my relationships with my friends has tailed off.

"They thought I was crazy when I got engaged," says Chris.

Chris says that it became impossible to fit his old friends into his married life. "I'd say my friends are jealous and mad because I don't come by as often as I did," he says. "My friends got mad when I chose my wife over them, and I don't think they understand that when you marry somebody your wife comes first."

Chris says he thinks "friends have a tendency to criticize you in terms of the relationship, so they feel superior. But hopefully in their hearts they're happy for you."

"We've got a couple married friends now," Chris adds. "That's something we've talked about, and we decided we need to have some people in our lives who don't react first and foremost to our relationship, but want to be our friends, as we are, together. It's sad when people's roles in our lives are reduced, but we can't let anyone undermine our lives."

Among those in a relationship, satisfaction was about 3 percent higher for each couple they regularly socialized with. (Cox 2001)

Your Goals Are a Living Thing

Goals have to evolve with you. They should be neither absurdly out of reach nor easily within reach. In either case, your motivation will be stalled by the uselessness of your goals.

Instead, keep your goals far enough away that you need to keep trying, but close enough that you can someday reach them.

IN 1978, KUMIKO Watanuki had her career goal set on eventually running the Iranian division of AT&T. Then revolution engulfed the country. She found herself forced out of the country, and forced to start over in the New York office, without any path for the future mapped out.

She set out to create a new career plan, and she capitalized on the advantages of being back in the United States. "I had the chance now to pursue a master's degree that the company would pay for, and I had access to company personnel I never could have met working half a world away," Kumiko says.

Advancement to the upper echelon of the company did not seem likely, however, and Kumiko realized that her international experience could be put to better use. Today, she runs a company that advises on international trade matters.

"I worked with a five-year plan of what I needed to do and what I wanted to accomplish. I've followed it, even though I had to take some detours, and I'm right where I want to be. I made my career plan an integral part of my life," Kumiko says.

More than seven out of ten Olympic athletes who won gold actually felt that their victory hurt their motivation for future training and weakened their ability to compete. (Jackson, Mayocchi, and Dover 1998)

Limit Yourself to Thinking About One Subject As You Go to Sleep

---

If you let your thoughts shoot around from one subject to another as you try to go to sleep, you can create an almost endless catalog of problems. With all these problems, you'll ask yourself, how can I possibly sleep? Tonight, as you are brushing your teeth or preparing for bed, come up with something you'd like to think about when you slip under the covers. If other thoughts start to intrude, guide yourself back to the original subject.

IMAGINE THAT YOU put your head down and try to sleep. You think about how much junk mail you get each day. Not only does it waste time, it also creates garbage. There's so much garbage. How can people throw out so much stuff? They say the landfills are nearly full. Where will the garbage go then? What will the environment be like for the next generation? Will the earth survive?

Dr. Morgan Edison warns that many people allow their presleep thoughts to drift like this. Here a minor annoyance leads to concerns about the future of the planet. And those concerns race around, causing stress instead of relaxation.

Too many thoughts, even if they don't lead to such drastic topics as the fate of the earth, are unsettling and make it much harder to sleep. When our thoughts bounce in and out, each idea backed by another, the stream of ideas makes us more on edge and less ready to close our eyes, shut off our brain for the day, and fall blissfully to sleep.

Shifting between presleep thoughts was found to be related to difficulty in sleeping and lower sleep quality, which, in turn, were related to unhappiness. Better sleepers are 6 percent more satisfied with their lives than average sleepers and 25 percent more satisfied than poor sleepers. (Peters, Joireman, and Ridgway 2005)

Express Yourself in What You Do

Do something today that reflects who you are, what you are capable of, what you care about. Whether it is at work, at home, for pay or for free, do something that shows you. We need to see evidence of our abilities; we need to see evidence of our relevance. Give yourself plenty of evidence of what you can do, and you will not doubt your abilities to do anything.

LARRY BRODY WROTE for numerous televisions shows including *Baretta, Barnaby Jones, Diagnosis Murder, Hawaii Five-O, The Six Million Dollar Man,* and *Walker, Texas Ranger.*

But one of the greatest joys of his work on television shows was working with other writers, particularly those just starting out. "I loved to help new colleagues grow into the role of being a writer," Larry says.

Larry decided he wanted to go into a semiretirement away from the stress of Hollywood life. From his Arkansas ranch he's organized a variety of opportunities for young writers to have their work critiqued, including contests for scripts and short films. Larry offers feedback based on his understanding of the fundamentals of writing. "If you've got the pacing and the rhythm, you've got half of it. If you have that, and something you want to share, you're just about there," he says.

The point of Larry's efforts is to nurture talent. "It's all about dreams—about making dreams come true," he says. In fact, at this point he takes more satisfaction from contributing to other writers than he does from writing himself. "I'd rather teach other people to put it together than do anything else in the business," he says.

People who felt they had an outlet for self-expression were 19 percent more likely to feel confident about themselves and 18 percent more likely to feel satisfied with their lives. (Christiansen 2000)

Hostility Hurts You

Positive connections between people are a source of mental and physical well-being. Negative feelings toward those around you are a source of mental and physical strain. Realize that your anger will hurt you more than it will hurt the target of your ire.

"MAYBE REAL MEN should eat quiche. They might live longer," says philosophy professor Sam Keen. In the name of better health, Sam argues for a male makeover that replaces violence, materialism, and power with peace, spirituality, and cooperation.

"We still are raised primarily in terms of warriors," Sam says. "Potency is the mark of a man, but that is a cultural identity that may make us sick with stress."

In his research, Sam became immersed in the relationship between spirituality and health. Because of what he learned, Sam encourages men to define a sense of self that is independent of cultural expectations. "The more we try to impose our vision on everyone," he says, "the more disappointed we become. That will sicken us."

Sam says too many men adopt values and behaviors that traditionally have been associated with them. He calls for men to "create their own stories" instead of believing the hand-me-down myths about them. "We are biologically aggressive animals, but aggression is different from hostility," he says. "'Aggressive' means we are energetic beings, and we have to do something with that energy. That energy can be channeled toward making peace as easily as waging war."

Doctors found that people with high levels of hostility were 6 percent more likely to suffer from heart disease. (Brown University 2002)

Changing Jobs Doesn't Change You

Transitions intimidate us because everything seems so different. But even as our surroundings change, we don't change. We need some stability in our lives to be able to function. When you undertake new things, rely on the stability of who you are to provide you with comfort and confidence.

AMY IS A career counselor who sees people changing jobs every day.

She also sees people fall into transition anxiety all the time. "It's like sending a five-year-old off to the first day of kindergarten. 'What's it going to be like?' 'What will happen to me?' The fears some people have would be funny if they weren't so real," Amy says.

Amy focuses her clients' attention on the one thing that doesn't change with a career move: themselves.

"Some people lose all sense of proportion, and really think everything in their world will change," Amy says. "Some look at that change as positive, as if all their old bad habits will go away. I compare changing jobs to changing relationships. You wouldn't just change relationships to solve your infidelity problem, because you would just bring the problem with you. And you can't just change jobs to make yourself into a new person: you'll be the same wherever you work, and work will be what you make of it wherever you go."

Nearly everyone feels some anxiety when starting a new job. However, people who focus their attention on their identity rather than on their uncertain surroundings feel less stress and report becoming comfortable in their new position in half as much time. (Childs 1998)

Share What You Know

There are things you know that other people would love to know and that you would enjoy sharing. Seek the opportunity to share what you know, and you will be rewarded with an opportunity to focus your attention on your abilities and accomplishments. Plus, you will have helped someone in the process.

THE CALLER MIGHT say they are from the credit-card company, or a utility, or a store. They will say there has been a problem: maybe some information has been lost or the computer malfunctioned. Can you just confirm some information on your credit file one more time?

As Rick explains to people in his California hometown, the calls are a scam meant to allow thieves to find out crucial information so that they can ultimately get credit in your name. "These companies already have all your information. And if they didn't, they wouldn't call and ask you for it," Rick explains.

Rick serves as a volunteer helping his local police department keep people informed about some of the sneakiest crimes out there. "Identity-theft issues are major, because you can be hurt without even knowing it. All your assets—your bank account, credit cards, your home—could be targeted," he warns.

Rick gives talks to groups and offers tips not only about the latest scams but about how to protect yourself and what to do if your identity is stolen. "The most important thing is to be proactive. Anyone who gets access to your credit is going to try to create as much damage as possible as fast as possible," Rick says.

Researchers studying people in their sixties have found that those who said they were in a mentoring type of relationship were 29 percent more likely to see meaning in their lives. (Van Handel Eagles 1999)

Home Is Where Accidents Happen

Our homes are comforting to us. It is where we spend most of our time. It is where we feel safest. But because of its role in our lives, it is also where the threat of accidental injuries is highest. Look through your house closely, and consider the potential accidents you could avoid in your home with some precautionary steps.

AS PATTY APPROACHED the front door of her home after completing a few errands, she heard the screech of smoke detectors. Horrified, she realized the electric Christmas candle had fallen from the front window onto the sofa, which was smoldering. She raced inside for the fire extinguisher but was too late. Once the drapes ignited, there was nothing for her to do but run out and dial 911.

"As soon as I got outside, the living-room windows blew out from the heat," she recalls. "Within fifteen minutes, the fire caused a quarter of a million dollars' worth of damage. I stood there and watched while the house I'd lived in for two decades was destroyed.

"I realized how slim the margin was from this fire being deadly. If it had happened at night, my whole family would have been in the house. If we didn't have smoke detectors, we might never have made it." Indeed, most fire-related fatalities occur in homes without smoke detectors.

After her home was finally rebuilt, Patty made some changes: "More smoke detectors, a sprinkler system, and no more electric candles."

A study found that 20,000 Americans die annually due to accidents within their homes, and another 7 million suffer injuries in their homes. Meanwhile, 56 percent of Americans said they had not made a single effort to make their homes safer. (University of North Carolina 2002a)

Take Off Your Blinders

Perspective is a powerful force. From a young age we are taught to have certain expectations, and those expectations influence how we see the world. Nobody would rationally choose to limit their aspirations, deny themselves opportunities, and misjudge other people's talents based on a set of stereotypes. But that is just what we do without even thinking about it, because stereotypes alter our view of the world.

IN NORTHERN NEW Hampshire, the Women's Rural Entrepreneurial Network (WREN) is helping women make an income from home.

WREN's members run the gamut from women selling handmade crafts in their spare time to women offering professional services such as graphic design and bookkeeping full-time.

WREN's director, Natalie Woodroofe, says the group helps bring women together who otherwise might be isolated and discouraged.

Natalie says WREN's members feel empowered to succeed and are more likely to overcome the skepticism that rural women working from home face when they try to make a living. "These women get more than their share of discouragement from people who act like they are seven-year-olds selling lemonade in their front yard," Natalie says.

Instead, WREN connects these work-at-home women with a network of women of all ages and professions. "There are business managers or owners who donate their time to WREN," Natalie adds. "WREN crosses all barriers—economic, cultural, educational—so that women can see their capabilities and their connections with each other."

Natalie says that "women who are creating and supporting themselves should feel good about what they do, and WREN helps make that happen."

People who are prone to use stereotypes in assessing themselves and others are 39 percent more likely to believe that opportunities are limited for others and themselves. (Frome 1999)

Smell Healthy

Our senses communicate to our brain whether we should be in a state of alarm or a state of calm. Even when we are in distress in our lives, soothing our senses helps to soothe our systems. Surround yourself with pleasant smells when you are feeling ill or stressed, and your system will be calmed.

BEFORE A MAGNETIC resonance imaging (MRI) exam, David, an MRI technologist, brings out his secret weapons.

He displays a black case with an eclectic collection of CDs: Beethoven, James Taylor, Yanni, Frank Sinatra, the Eurythmics, Alanis Morissette. As you lie on the scanning table, he pops your choice into a CD player. Soon the music wafts through your headphones. Then he covers your eyelids with an aromatherapy eye pillow scented with a few drops of cucumber or lavender essential oil.

Peacefully, patients are introduced to the MRI process.

The music may not completely drown out the machine's loud bangs, but it and the scent may help you tune out the stress and anxiety during what some consider an unsettling and claustrophobic experience.

An increasing number of health-care providers say they're using these and other methods to help patients banish anxiety during diagnostic tests and before surgery. His co-workers on the radiology staff have found that to be true, David says. The number of patients who cannot tolerate an MRI has decreased since the music option was offered several years ago. That number has dropped further since the department began providing aromatherapy.

A study of women in labor found that aromatherapy—surrounding the patient with pleasant smells—helped them relax and feel in control. Over 80 percent of women rated the aromatherapy effective as helping them through even the most painful moments of labor. (Oxford University 2002a)

Music Can Bring Us Together

Think about a situation in which a couple is on the brink of being irritated with each other. Maybe they had a hard day, or maybe one said something that could be taken the wrong way. They sit uncomfortably—the silence between them magnifying the tension. And then, one of them puts on their favorite album. The music enters their thoughts. The tension dissipates, and both partners are put in mind of shared joys and good times.

"WHEN YOU'RE OLD, people think you've either lost your nut or you've got some special knowledge. Here's what I have: 'You have to give and take,'" says ninety-three-year-old Herbert. "And obey the golden rule."

"And forgive each other," added Elsie, his ninety-year-old wife.

The couple met at a local dance. The attraction was immediate, but their courtship lasted more than a year. "We went to a lot of dances," Elsie says.

They spent their entire lives trying to make a living on their small Missouri farm. "A lot of our neighbors went bankrupt trying," Herbert says.

For many years, their home had no electricity. "We could only spend a nickel once a year for ice cream," Elsie says.

"I tell a lot of people how we had it, and they don't believe it," her husband agrees.

"I always had a piano, though," Elsie recalls. "And he played the violin. And you know what? I'd start playing and he'd start playing, and the next thing you know we're teenagers at a dance again. It never fails."

Though things weren't easy, their marriage was happy because, Edie says, "we needed each other, and we had fun."

Exposing a couple to music of their choice increased feelings of cooperation and caring in seven in ten people. (Housker 2001)

You Are Not in This Alone

The American Dream. The American work ethic. The American pioneer spirit. If you listen to the slogans, you can't help but think it's every man for himself, and every person's success or failure is completely their own. Thinking this way and feeling this way feeds a certain sense of desperation. "The outcome is riding on me, everything that happens, or doesn't happen, is because of me." But every step of the way, there have been people to protect us and teach us. And for all the power of the American individualistic spirit, no one, not even the most independent of the pioneers, has succeeded alone.

DECADES AGO, MILWAUKEE'S King Drive was a thriving retail center.

Then hard times fell on the surrounding neighborhood and the businesses that lined King Drive.

Today, the street is making a comeback, spurred by entrepreneurs who are working together to help each other and to help the community. Business owners have formed an association and have worked to have sites on the street declared historic buildings.

They also offer training and loans to new King Drive business owners, because, as Lennie Mosely, who moved her already established business to King Drive, explains, "We want to have more of a stake in the community. Our dreams are happening here.

"We make it clear to everybody who gives this place a try: 'You are not in this by yourself. We're in this together.'"

One urban-planning researcher says of their efforts, "From what I've seen around the country, King Drive stands out as one of the best examples of inner-city redevelopment."

People who acknowledge the interdependent nature of life, the importance of human connections, and our collective existence were twice as likely to consider themselves successful. (Carpenter 2000)

Value the Multiple Uses of Aspirin

The most common headache relief provider until it was displaced by ibuprofen and acetaminophen, aspirin reduces our susceptibility to blood clots and has been linked to a reduced risk for heart disease and Alzheimer's disease.

"ASPIRIN CAN DEFINITELY be called a wonder drug, ranked right up there with penicillin. But it is a drug," says Dr. Thomas Cassidy.

"Historically, aspirin was first used as a pain reliever, but why it worked was not known. Now we know that the body reacts to injury by releasing hormonelike substances called prostaglandins, which cause inflammation, redness, swelling, and subsequent pain. Aspirin blocks the enzyme responsible for production of prostaglandins. Aspirin has also been used for decreasing fever and inflammation," Dr. Cassidy says.

"Today, we appreciate the fact that aspirin reduces blood clotting," he adds. "This was first thought of as a potentially negative side effect, but it is really a tremendous benefit. Decreased clotting aids in the prevention and treatment of strokes.

"More recently, researchers noticed that people who took even small amounts of aspirin regularly had a decreased risk of heart attacks from coronary artery disease. This was attributed to the effect on clotting. It now appears that reduced inflammation is also an important way in which aspirin decreases heart attacks.

"In fact, my advice is, if you are a woman over fifty or a man over forty, taking aspirin each day is a valuable step in reducing your susceptibility to major disease," Dr. Cassidy says.

Elderly people who took aspirin daily for more than two years showed a 55 percent lower rate of dementia. Taking aspirin every day reduced the rate of heart attacks by 44 percent and of certain kinds of cancer by 50 percent. (Mayo Clinic 2002a)

Make Your Decisions for Positive Reasons

Too often in relationships we ask ourselves, "What's to be lost if I make this decision?" instead of "What's to be gained?" This pattern can lead to the continuation of unsatisfying situations because of a fear that things might get worse. Make your decisions based on getting what you do want, not avoiding what you don't.

NOT TOO LONG ago, Ali was giddy. She'd met a great guy, and she was so confident in the relationship's future that she moved in with him after just a few weeks of dating. The couple was engaged a few months later, and soon married. "We knew that we were going to be together forever," Ali says.

"It was good at first," she says. But Ali says she was too free-spirited to fit into her husband's orderly existence: "Me being in the same space with somebody, it just became like putting two dogs in a cage together."

Still, the cage, as she calls it, was comfortable for a while.

Even as she thought they were both unhappy, neither sought a change. "We had just bought a house—so that made it hard to walk away," Ali says. "Then, I didn't look forward to saying to everyone I knew and my family that I'd made a big mistake. Especially when I knew some of them had been shaking their heads from the start."

They continued living together for six months after she had decided the relationship was broken. Then she gave up. Ali says, "I've learned you can't keep a relationship alive merely for convenience's sake."

In a study of those who in their relationships had faced feelings of betrayal, people who continued in the relationship for fearful or negative reasons were overwhelmingly unsatisfied with the relationship (61 percent) or had discontinued the relationship six months later (24 percent). (Roloff, Soule, and Carey 2001)

Think About Who You Ought to Be

The more you direct yourself toward a fantasy life, the less satisfied you will be with who you are, and the more frustrated you will become as you fail to attain the fantasy. The more you direct yourself toward a better, more fulfilling life, the more you can actually lead a better, more fulfilling life.

LISA WORKS IN communications, and she thinks of herself as the second Darren on the old television show *Bewitched*. Every other day there is a different person doing her job, and no one seems to notice.

Lisa shares her job, working every other day, while her job partner at the company takes the other days.

Lisa asked for the arrangement so that she could spend more time with her child, but she recognizes the challenge of the shared job. "It's a relay race when most of us are used to running by ourselves. It requires tremendous cooperation, organization, and mutual respect," she says.

Although thrilled when her boss approved the work-sharing plan, Lisa acknowledges that "every fantasy has a reality. The choice comes down to time or money, and you have to make a decision as to which matters more."

Cutting her salary has made things a little tight at home, and she is concerned that her potential for advancement may be hurt when she returns to working full-time; but for her, the decision was clearly the right thing to do: "I have a healthier perspective on life, and a healthier family life, and nothing matters more to me than that."

People who are focused on the "ideal" life they could lead are 34 percent more likely to be anxious and self-conscious about their lives, while people who are focused on the life they "ought" to lead are more caring about other people in their lives and are actually 21 percent more oriented toward achieving in their careers. (Bybee, Luthar, and Zigler 1997)

Noise Matters

The requirements of life such as food, shelter, and safety must also include avoiding oppressively loud noise. Whether in the workplace or at home, prolonged exposure to uncomfortable levels of noise will affect your ability to think, your ability to remember, your disposition, and your overall health.

YOU'RE SITTING IN your car at a traffic light as you shift into unwind at the end of the workday. Suddenly your vehicle is vibrating from a deafening sound. Your shoulders immediately rise to meet the lobes of your ears. Your heart pounds. And then you turn to see if your partners in traffic have also hunched down in survival mode. Then you see him: the person in the booming car next to you, bopping to the thundering reverberations.

Enter Ted Rueter. No, he's not the fellow conducting the car concert next to you. He is the sound of one hand clapping. The founder of Noise Free America, he is a mild-mannered political science professor at Tulane University. He walks softly and carries a loud message on low volume. Professor Rueter gets riled up about boom cars and leaf blowers. He's concerned about your health—and the quality of your environment.

Noise, says the antinoise crusader, lowers sex drive, causes sleep deprivation and depression, "harms cognitive development and language acquisition," and results in hearing loss. Loud noise causes our heart to beat faster, our pulse rate to go up, our digestive juices to slow down, our blood pressure to rise—"all related to the stress of noise."

Professor Rueter warns, "We are becoming a nation oblivious to noise while suffering the consequences."

Researchers have found that workers in noisy offices experienced significantly higher levels of stress and made 40 percent fewer attempts to solve a difficult problem they were presented with. (Cornell University 2002b)

Work on Your Own Terms

The line of work you have chosen either suits you or it doesn't. No amount of trying to force a round personality into a square job will make work that conflicts with your identify meet your needs.

EVA HAS BEEN a waitress at a restaurant in Milwaukee for twenty-five years. "I've always felt that everybody's job is important," Eva says. "When I step out on the floor, everything else goes away. This is what I do, and I enjoy it very much."

Eva says the work is similar to any frontline position in a company: "It's a sales job, like selling clothing or anything else. I'm the person you meet, not the chef or the manager."

Eva grew up in what is now Slovakia and came to the United States not knowing a word of English. She learned the language one word at a time using flash cards and eventually earned a college degree. She had thoughts about going to graduate school, but she didn't want to stop waitressing.

"I started to work as a waitress when I started going through school, and I really liked it," she says. "I like the job, and it suits my needs.

"You realize that, coming here from a fairly poor country, you don't need everything. Just enough. I'm very grateful to be here. My needs and wants are simple."

But Eva doesn't recommend waiting on tables unless it is something you really want to do. "It's like any job," she says. "You just have to love it. Otherwise, you are miserable."

How interested people are in their work, how much control they feel over their work, and how much support they feel they get from their employer are collectively nineteen times more important in predicting job satisfaction than are people's family life situations. (Goulet and Singh 2002)

Never Let Faults Stand for the Whole

When asked about their partners, people in long-term relationships don't bring up a long list of complaints. It's not that their partners are perfect, but their tendency isn't to dwell on faults. In fact, people in long-term relationships not only spend much more time thinking about the good traits of their partners but also tend to see redeeming features even in the faults.

RODDY CLEARY, A Unitarian minister, has performed dozens of civil-union ceremonies since a historic bill went into effect in Vermont allowing gay and lesbian couples to have their relationships recognized by the state. Her husband, William, also performs civil-union ceremonies.

Roddy and William describe themselves as "wildly, madly, insanely in love." Married for thirty-three years, they see their role as helping other couples come together and demonstrate their love. "Uniting couples in love strengthens our society. Gender is incidental," Roddy says.

Roddy's interpretation of the Scriptures makes her one of the few clergy members willing to perform civil-union ceremonies. She tells participants, "To be able to share in another's joy is what heaven is about."

Roddy sees both her own marriage and her participation in other unions as the ultimate expression "of seeing the good in people.

"I received a letter from a man who didn't want his daughter to marry another woman. It says, 'Your sense of spirituality, your obvious pleasure in addressing our daughter's spirituality, enhanced our joy.' And I think, maybe for the first time, he saw some good in his daughter's marriage."

People in long-term relationships spent five times as much time talking in response to a question about their partner's positive qualities as they did talking about negative qualities, and tended to qualify negative comments by explaining away their importance. (Murray and Holmes 1999)

Care

Whether at home or at work, people who find their lives fulfilling care about those around them. They engage themselves in those around them, actively concerning themselves with their lives, concerns, interests, and well-being.

WHEN HIS TEXTILE mill, Malden Mills, burned down in December 1995, it was a terrible blow for Aaron Feuerstein.

He'd invested heavily, both with his money and with his life, in keeping his business alive and thriving despite foreign competition, which paid its workers inhuman wages and could therefore undercut his prices.

When the architects, contractors, and accountants tallied up the costs of rebuilding, Aaron worried about whether the business could go on. But the more he thought about the business, the more he thought about the more than two thousand people who worked for him. People who came in every morning and worked hard all day, turning out a quality product that had brought in profits even when everybody else said it couldn't be done.

Aaron made a decision then that not only would he rebuild his mill, but he would keep paying his employees while the mill was closed during the months of construction work ahead. Tears of sorrow at what had happened to the plant, and what would happen to them, turned to tears of joy on his workers' faces.

Today, the plant is up and running, and Malden Mills workers are, according to Aaron, "about the most loyal and hardworking people you could ever meet."

Eight in ten CEOs report that a healthy family life is crucial to a productive business life and that the same key skill, "interpersonal engagement"—the capacity to express concern and interest in those around them—is crucial to both home and work. (Henderson 1999)

Don't Accept Television's Picture of the World

Watch television for any length of time, whether it's the news or a prime-time show, and you will inevitably come to the conclusion that virtually everyone is either very rich or about to die a horrible, bloody death. These images affect us more than we know. We fear that the awful events on television will happen to us, and we are frustrated that the nearly universal wealth we see on television hasn't reached us yet. Separate what you see from what you know to be real. Base your expectations on reality, not television.

FOR A THOUSAND generations, the Gwich'in tribe lived in northern Alaska in nearly complete isolation from outside cultures. Tribal members were completely self-sufficient, surviving on skills taught to them by their parents and elders.

In 1980, one of the tribe's leaders acquired a television.

Members of the tribe describe the event as the beginning of an addiction. Soon the native customs were ignored to maximize TV-watching time. One researchers says of the tribe's experience, "For these natives, like anyone else, television is a cultural nerve gas. It's odorless, painless, tasteless, and deadly."

What happened to the Gwich'in traditions that had existed for thousands of years? In the words of one tribe member, "Television made us wish we were something else. It taught us greed and waste, and now everything that we were is gone."

Television changes our view of the world and can encourage us to develop highly unrealistic and often damaging conclusions that serve to reduce our life satisfaction by up to 50 percent. (Jeffres and Dobos 1995)

Don't Wait to Start Moving in the Right Direction

We will often continue down the path we are on regardless of whether we find it rewarding or even acceptable. Don't wait for the moment that shakes you out of your routine; work on making your life as fulfilling as you want right now.

HE WAS A prominent Texas surgeon. He appeared in television ads for his medical clinic, smiling as he said, "We treat you like family."

When she first met the surgeon, Colleen was awed by him. After a few dates, she says, "he told me that he wanted me to quit my job, that he loved me, and that he would support me. And that everything would be great." When he proposed, Colleen accepted.

Colleen says her new husband quickly became more and more controlling, insisting she drop plans for college and demanding to know her whereabouts all the time.

After a separation, the two eventually reconciled, and there was new hope for the marriage with the birth of a daughter. However, the relationship instead began spiraling into violence.

The pattern continued for more than a year, she says: "I realize now, of course, that I was indulging this fantasy that he would change."

Colleen eventually divorced the doctor and successfully sued him for inflicting physical abuse. "I'm stronger now than what I ever was with him," concludes Colleen.

In the aftermath of major hurricanes that level or flood out entire towns, researchers have found that people tend to critically examine their lives, which produces increases of 25 percent in marriage rates, as people decide to take their relationships to a higher level, and increases of 32 percent in divorce rates, as people examine their relationships and find them unfulfilling. (Cohan and Cole 2002)

Failure Is Not to Try

You can never fail if you don't bother to try. This, of course, is the ultimate failure, for it means you can never make progress toward your goals.

JEFF HOWARD IS a school psychologist who studies how we teach youngsters and how they learn. He says most school systems informally break their student body into three groups: the very smart, the kind of smart, and the kind of dumb.

By the time they reach the sixth grade, those consigned to the kind of dumb group are already well versed in the low expectations educators have for them.

"We put up barriers to these children in middle school, barriers we don't expect them to climb over," Jeff says.

Jeff argues every student has the capacity to learn more—that studies of the learning capacity of the average four-year-old are more optimistic than the treatment the "kind of dumb" middle schooler typically receives.

The real danger in grouping students into these categories is the biggest lesson they teach: For the top group, anything is possible, so never stop trying. For the bottom group, nothing is possible, so don't bother trying. Indeed, bottom-group students mock those of their classmates who care or try to succeed.

Jeff's experimental solution involves putting students of all levels together and placing clear expectations and rewards in front of all of them. Early results have shown that all students, from all three levels, improve their test scores when expectations are increased.

When asked to describe significant regrets in their lives, more than eight out of ten people focused on actions they did not take rather than actions they did. In other words, they focused on things they failed to do rather than things they failed at doing. (Ricaurte 1999)

If You Don't Believe, No One Else Will

Sometimes we look to others to convince us of what we want to believe. But the people around you will most likely mirror your feelings—showing you fear when you show fear, demonstrating confidence when you demonstrate confidence. You can't rely on others to convince you, because they will rely on you to convince them.

PAUL GONZALES GREW up in a very poor Los Angeles neighborhood.

He remembers the occasional career day when successful people would visit his school and tell the students a little about what they did. Paul says those visits did little for him, because he could never see himself in their place.

As he grew up, he witnessed a barrage of violence, culminating in the murder of a cousin. Paul decided that he had to make a change: "That day, I made a promise to myself. I would never make sorrow for others. I would make joy for what I accomplished."

As a fourteen-year-old, Paul turned away from the neighborhood gangs and began training with the local police athletic league. "I knew I had to do something for myself," Paul explains about a regimen that began with 5 A.M. workouts. Ultimately he chose boxing as his sport, and he set his sights on the Olympics.

In 1984, Paul made the U.S. Olympic boxing team and went on to win a gold medal. He's now a guest at career days in Los Angeles, and he tells students that the most important thing they can learn is this: "You can do anything you want, but you have to believe in yourself first."

People were five times more likely to be optimistic about another person's goals if they thought the person was optimistic himself or herself. Less significant factors included the person's personal experiences and the overall likelihood of the outcome. (Werneck De Almeida 1999)

Don't Let Negativity Build

When there is anger and disappointment in a family, it is almost inevitable that it will build on itself. When a family member is disruptive, seek not only to stop the behavior but to solve the problem at its root.

ACTING IS THEIR family business. Their parents ran an acting school when they were young. Eric Roberts and his sisters Lisa and Julia grew up together, imagining a future as actors, which they all achieved to varying degrees of acclaim. Now, Eric and his sisters are not on speaking terms.

"We disagree on a couple of key family issues, as every family does. But because we're famous we're under a microscope, so it gets compounded. It's just part of the package, and it's an unfortunate part of the package," Eric says.

Eric admits he was less than an ideal brother years ago. He says his sisters "decided I was more trouble than I was worth, and I can't really blame them." But the worst part of it for Eric is that each family problem gave way to a bigger one. "What started out as a disappointment turned into a conflict which turned into a war. Each step was putting us in a worse position," Eric recalls.

Eric laments that he has not had any opportunity to apologize and heal the rift in his family. "I've tried to contact them many times, and they ignored me," he says. "So I stopped. I would like for a reunion to happen. And if it doesn't it's all our loss, and if it does it's all our gain."

Psychologists have observed that family members who are angry with each other are six times more likely to expand a conflict into unrelated areas than they are after the initial anger subsides. (Hoeveler 1999)

See a New Way

W hen the easy answers have been tried and the problem remains, the time is ripe for your creative powers. Be willing to look at things in a new way, think about them with a fresh perspective, and tap the hidden ideas within your brain.

GERRY WAS AN executive with a major financial company. Every day was stressful and long and featured a brutal commute. "At some point you have to ask yourself why you are doing this," he says.

Offered the opportunity to take a dramatic pay cut to head his hometown's YMCA, Gerry jumped at the chance.

His commute is now three minutes long, and his days are stress-free. But more important than those things, Gerry says, is the fact that the career switch has given him the chance to make a difference in his community: "Every day I'm thinking about how to serve people through this organization. A good decision doesn't shift the marginal return rate on some unseen transaction; a good decision serves a person who lives right down the street.

"In the corporate world I saw it as important for me to do as well as I could do financially," Gerry says. "But now I realize it's important for me to be closer to home, to do something that really resonates with me today in terms of my values.

"I realize this doesn't match the corporate world in pay, but neither can the corporate world feed my spirit as much as this does," he says.

Among those experiencing low life satisfaction, the willingness to think creatively about their problems was associated with an 11 percent shorter duration of negative feelings. (Zhou and George 2001)

Remember the Drugs We Tend to Forget

What is the single most popular drug in the world? You might make fifty wrong guesses before you remember caffeine. Caffeine use is so widespread in coffee, tea, chocolate, and soda that we conveniently overlook its status as a drug. In low doses, caffeine can have positive effects, and for that reason it is used in some pain relievers. In high doses, however, caffeine can not only interfere with sleep but increase blood pressure.

IT SEEMS HARMLESS enough. A citrus-flavored powder packed with vitamins, minerals, and a jolt of caffeine. You mix it with water or fruit juice, drink it, and you're off to seize the day. But because of its popularity with high school athletes, use of the drink has generated a stir among parents and coaches.

"Caffeine is a stimulant. High concentrations are banned by the NCAA and the International Olympic Committee," says one concerned parent. "This product contains five times the caffeine of a cola drink."

Another says, "The biggest danger is that these products can be seen as some kind of magic bullet. Young people, like anyone else, are looking for an edge in sports. They think something they can buy and take will make them better. And in this case, you're sprinkling it in juice, so they think it must be food for them. But there is no evidence to show this will help them, and there have been good reasons that respected sports organizations across the world have banned excessive caffeine consumption in athletes."

The majority of scientific evidence shows that, for a healthy adult, moderate quantities of caffeine (250 to 350 milligrams per day—the equivalent of about three cups of coffee) pose no significant health risks. However, a link between higher amounts of caffeine and certain heart problems such as arrhythmias has been reported. (University of Texas 2002)

The Pieces of Your Life Must Fit Together

Your two favorite foods might be delightful separately but terrible in combination with each other. We know that, and we make decisions on what makes a good meal based on that. Ultimately, your career and your relationship are not two separate parts of your life, but two forces that combine to make your life. Seek not two ideals that would never fit together, but two compatible situations that will make your life work.

JANE IS A coach. A life coach. Based in Portland, Oregon, she helps clients throughout the country reach their goals in everything from efficient use of time to career planning to life satisfaction.

She holds weekly meetings in person, on the phone, or by email with her clients. Jane discusses seeking fulfillment and balance in such matters as career, family, health, and hobbies. Jane boasts that the right coach "may not help you find anything you weren't going to find eventually, but a coach can take the learning curve down from forty years to two years." Jane says that comes from two factors: "helping people find their focus" and "highlighting the future, and what it has to offer."

Despite enjoying the work immensely, Jane says, she realized there was something missing: "I spent my time guiding people to their own fulfillment, and then woke up one day and realized I wasn't heading toward mine." She evaluated where she was and, with the help of her own coach, decided to seek a better balance between her work and her personal life.

"I help people pursue their dreams; but to keep doing that, I have to pursue mine too," Jane says.

More than seven in ten professionals report that their job has been in the way of a satisfying personal life at some point in their career. (Gilbert and Walker 2001)

You'll Work Harder If You Feel Wanted

It might sound small, but it's true. We work harder and better when we feel appreciated. Money, prestige, and all the other aspects of work we benefit from will still be compromised if we do not think that those we work for care about us.

WAINWRIGHT INDUSTRIES OF Missouri says its average employee generated fifty-five ideas per year to improve the company's production of automotive and aerospace parts.

Wainwright's chairman, Don Wainwright, credits his company's attitude toward employees for fostering creativity: "In most organizations, the managers operate like parents who make the rules and then administer punishments and rewards. The nonmanagers play a corollary role of children who have to be good and do what mom and dad say ... or else." Wainright, he says, "adopted a 'People First Policy' that avoids this parent trap and instead encourages every employee to speak up when they have a better idea, instead of either making the suggestion to a superior, who would then steal credit as the idea worked its way up the line, or, ultimately, not saying anything at all."

The policy has been a huge success, with Don Wainright crediting it for a 35 percent drop in production costs and a 91 percent drop in customer rejection rates. It also helped bring home the coveted Malcolm Baldridge National Quality Award.

Lower-management workers who felt like they were appreciated by superiors were 52 percent less likely to look for a different job. (Jones 2000)

Do You Work in a Sick Building?

Buildings with inadequate ventilation can trap poor-quality air inside while recirculating viruses and contaminants throughout. If you regularly feel ill at work, find out everything you can about your building's ventilation system.

"THERE'S NOT A lot you can do in a modern building with windows that don't open," laments Joe Stearns, who has both worked in and studied the air quality of office buildings. "We got too good at sealing off a building. We thought it would be wonderful for reducing heating and cooling costs. But it is also wonderful for trapping things we don't want inside the building."

Joe says the culprits include chemical contaminants from indoor sources such as adhesives, carpeting, upholstery, manufactured wood products, copy machines, pesticides, and cleaning agents that all emit volatile organic compounds. In low levels, these compounds can cause acute reactions in some people. However, high concentrations may lead to chronic health problems. Chemical contaminants from outdoor sources, such as vehicle exhaust, plumbing vents, and building exhausts, can also plague a building by entering through ill-placed air-intake vents.

"Your company should be monitoring the air quality in the building," Joe says. "If there is a problem, the company should be open about the condition and the steps being taken to resolve it.

"At the individual level, though, you can help the air quality in your office with plants. NASA did scientific research that proved foliage and flowering plants have the ability to clear the air of these pollutants and help with sick-building syndrome and improve indoor air quality."

Nearly 30 percent of office buildings worldwide have poor air quality. (World Health Organization 2001)

Show You Care, Even When It's Hard To

There is no more important time to demonstrate that you care, that you value your partner, than when difficulties arise. Even as you disagree, which you will, never fail to recognize and to show what matters most to you.

DURING GROUP RELATIONSHIP sessions, counselor Peter Dilliard explains that each person in a relationship must invest time, energy, and interest in the other one. "If you're not willing to invest in the people in your life, love will not grow. Investing in someone means caring about that person's feelings as part of your day-to-day life and understanding their needs," Peter says.

"The relationship investment involves sacrifice," Peter tells participants, "even though the word is not usually associated with relationships. Sacrifice is doing something you don't want to do because it will make the other person happy.

"No matter how hard it gets, you don't withdraw, emotionally disengage, and stop investing in the relationship," Peter says. "You can't be a rock and be loved. You must open up and be vulnerable. Love grows as you make the other person feel special and invest in the other person."

Peter draws some looks of disbelief when he declares, "If managed properly, conflict can bring a couple closer together." But he says that if you focus on the solution, not on the disagreement or who is at fault, "a conflict becomes a way of demonstrating commitment, love, and understanding. It becomes a way of demonstrating the strength of the relationship, not the weakness."

When couples experience conflict, they are 45 percent less likely to feel pessimistic about their relationship if they can recognize feelings of caring from their partner during the disagreement. (Ebesu Hubbard 2001)

Electric Brushing Is Easier, but Not Much Different

A re electric toothbrushes and other automatic devices worth the expense? If you would otherwise not do a thorough job of brushing with your manual toothbrush, the answer is yes. If you would otherwise brush for as long as and in the style recommended by your dentist, the answer is no.

DR. MARK HARRIS has a message for his dental patients and for everyone else: "Brushing your teeth is not like scrubbing your floors.

"Some people think that a stiff, hard brush applied with a vengeance is an effective approach, but plaque doesn't have to be scrubbed off, just reached," he says. "And a soft brush does less damage."

The most effective brushing is gentle, and is practiced often. "You would do yourself much more good brushing well after every meal than giving yourself the top-of-the-line automatic toothbrush and using it once a day," Dr. Harris says.

On the other hand, "some people are simply not going to listen to directions," Dr Harris says. "And just as they might scrub too hard and take the finish off their car, they can brush too hard and damage their teeth and gums. For those people, I recommend taking your car to a car wash and giving your teeth an automatic toothbrush."

But no matter what the brush shape or strokes per minute, preventing cavities and gum disease depends on all areas of the teeth getting cleaned. "Whatever toothbrush you use, you should make sure it enables you to reach everywhere in your mouth," Dr. Harris says.

Properly brushing and flossing manually is just as effective as using electric products. However, people such as those with arthritis, who have difficulty using manual products, benefit from the use of electric toothbrushes and electric flossing devices. (Mayo Clinic 2002d)

Avoid Roller-Coaster Emotions

Everybody likes some excitement in their world. But the heights of feeling good are usually followed by the depths of feeling bad. A successful life is not to be found in one exciting day—but in a steady, productive, fulfilling career.

TONY AND CARLA made it through the lean years. He was still in school. She worked hard to pay for their expenses and then came home and worked hard to cook meals, keep their home in order, and generally makes things as nice as she could for Tony.

"Back then," Carla remembers, "it was an uphill struggle, but it was our uphill struggle. And we just kept on going, with each other."

And now, degree in hand, Tony has reached new heights. Financial struggles are gone. In fact, most everything of their early married life is gone.

But instead of satisfaction, he rants against the fact that Carla hasn't become a new person to match the new person he is. Carla worries about what it means: "I don't want everything to change, I don't want to be a new person. I don't want to live every day anxious about whether I'm good enough or whether I'm going to do something that disappoints him again."

Tony tells her she ignored the part about marriage being for better not worse, and she's ruining the better.

Instead, Carla longs for the time "when our lives were steady. It was hard, but it was steady," she says.

Long-term studies of corporate leaders find that seven in ten of those who survive longest in their jobs downplay both the best and worst outcomes they experience and keep their feelings relatively steady. They have what psychologists call a "focus on an acceptable average," not on the extraordinary—which is useful because almost every day turns out to be more average than extraordinary. (Ingram 1998)

We Are All Much More Alike Than Different

When we think of people, we often focus on their differences. We see different groups, different religions, different ethnicities. We imagine that these different groups do things quite differently from us. But the struggles and hopes that characterize our notions of relationships are the same as those of countless others. Do not allow surface differences to overwhelm your acknowledgment of inner similarities.

BEV AND SIL face challenges that might overwhelm anyone. As a lesbian couple, they are not allowed to legally marry. Without being married, Bev, an American citizen, and Sil, who is from England, cannot obtain the family waiver that the U.S. government offers to provide citizenship to the foreign spouses of U.S. citizens.

"I do not know when I will see my beloved again, because our love is not respected by the laws of either of our countries," Bev says.

"As we all are painfully aware," she continues, "it doesn't have to be like that. Usually governments allow and even encourage binational couples by making immigration relatively simple for them. It is not too dramatic to say that we are actually being forced apart by our governments." Both Bev and Sil make extended visits to each other, but cannot legally stay in the other's country longer than six months.

"And yet, the truth of the matter is, the irony of all this is, we aren't any different than any other couple," Bev says. "We love, honor, and respect each other like any other couple should. We have arguments, get on each other's nerves sometimes, like any other couple, and we want nothing more than the same chance any other couple has to face up to the challenges of life and a relationship."

In how they viewed relationships, fears and feelings about relationships, and conceptions of ideal relationships, responses were similar across all ethnic groups in the United States. (LeSure-Lester 2001)

Value Practical Knowledge

E very year millions of young people finish school full of confidence
and self-importance, and arrive in the workplace only to find out
how much they don't know. Don't overlook the great importance of
the practical knowledge you have, and the importance of the practical
knowledge you can gain by learning every aspect of the things you do.

PATTY GRIFFIN SPENT years on the coffeehouse circuit, looking for any
chance to play her music for an audience.

The New England native was thrilled when she finally got her big
break, a contract with A&M Records.

She found herself a veteran producer and plunged head-first into the
studio to record. After an exhausting two months of studio work, she
had an album to play for the record company.

And they immediately rejected it.

Patty realized that it wasn't a rejection of her as much as a rejection
of the process that she had followed, one where her input was ignored.
"My voice got lost in the production," Patty says. "It became the producer's record, not mine. It was very far from the direction I wanted to go."

She wondered what would happen if she sent the record company
copies of her songs recorded in practice sessions, songs recorded without
a producer or a professional band. Despite the fact that some of the
songs were performed while Patty was sitting at a kitchen table, the
record company loved them as she had originally created them.

With her songs as she wanted them intact on the album, Patty
learned a lesson: "I knew better what I could do—how to bring my
voice, figuratively and literally, into a record."

Knowledge gained through workplace experience was six times more important than grades earned in school in predicting the job performance of
new employees. (Sternberg et al. 2000)

Guilt Is Bad for You

Wallowing in disappointment over something you did is not productive. Not only are you going to mentally exhaust yourself; you can also compromise your body's ability to ward off disease. Carrying the burden of disappointment in yourself or in others is something we choose to do—and something we would choose not to do if we had our health in mind.

"ONE THING THERE'S no shortage of is guilt," says Henry, a counselor who works with many people overburdened with the demands of career and family. "An average person can spend just about every minute of the day worrying about what they won't have time to do.

"Then you waste a good bit of the time you do have feeling bad about not having enough of it."

Henry recommends making a clear distinction between productive time and wasted time: "You need to separate out the time that is contributing neither to your home life nor to your work life—whether that's time wasted being inefficient or time wasted worrying—and maximize the use of your time for what matters."

Henry also advises us not to make promises we'll have trouble keeping: "If you say you are going to do something, you simply have to do it. Failing to do so will leave you deep in guilt. So be strategic about what you say you are going to do. Think about what you want to commit to, and be realistic about it.

"These kinds of things will cut down on the guilt you carry, which is the least productive thing you can do. It is a burden on your mental health and your physical health."

Feelings of guilt, according to a study, interfere with our bodies' production of the antibody immunoglobulin A, which protects against infection. (University of Hull 2002)

The Relationship Test: Are You Lonely?

There are countless qualities we seek in a partner, but the matters of true importance are few in number. The ultimate test of a relationship's health is a simple question: are you lonely? If you are in a relationship and unable to answer no, then the relationship is not meeting your most fundamental needs.

"IS THIS HOW I'm supposed to feel," Tonya remembers thinking to herself, "married but alone?"

Tonya's spouse worked long hours at the office, came home, and worked more hours there. When not working, he wanted time to himself. "He would say 'I need a few minutes here,' which meant don't bother him, don't ask him to do anything, or even be there with you," Tonya recalls.

"I realized that what we had on most days was not that different than if I was a hired hand. I do some things for you, I stay out of your way, I make no demands, I'm grateful for the occasional word of praise," she says.

Tonya gave up on waiting for him to notice the problem. "Subtlety was not getting me much of a response," she says. One day, after a series of long workdays followed by long worknights, and a growing feeling of complete invisibility, Tonya moved out. Though she went only a few miles away, her point had clearly been made.

Tonya's husband examined his habits, now put in stark relief based on what she'd done. He asked Tonya to forgive him for his thoughtlessness and pledged that he would seek to be her partner in all respects in the future. Two years later Tonya says, "I feel like I have a true partner now."

In studies of people in long-term committed relationships, more than a quarter of respondents admitted feeling lonely on a regular basis. Of those, only 8 percent thought their relationship was healthy. (Levine 2000)

Be Careful with Botox

Botox is everywhere in the headlines and news shows. The popular conception is that a quick and easy injection can take years off the appearance of your face. But Botox injection is a serious medical procedure that should not be considered without your doctor's input, and Botox should be administered only by a trusted physician.

THE NEW RAGE—the Botox party—may seem innocent fun for a group who wants to participate in this nonsurgical cosmetic procedure. But the chair of plastic surgery at the University of Texas Southwestern Medical Center at Dallas cautions that there can be unwanted consequences.

Dr. Rod Rohrich warns, "Botox should be used only by a qualified, trained physician. This procedure is not like applying an antiwrinkle cream. Botox is a drug, and there is a potential for complications."

Dr. Rohrich says, "Botox helps smooth out wrinkles around the eyes, forehead, and mouth by blocking the signal that causes the muscle to contract. One treatment generally lasts from three to four months.

"Some may not be good candidates for Botox," Dr. Rohrich warns. "Each potential patient should be evaluated individually."

Dr. Rohrich advises patients to be on the lookout for unscrupulous businesses that may dilute Botox and sell treatments for as little as $100: "If someone is quoting you an unreasonably low price, the serum may be watered down, and results will not last as long." He also warns against Botox parties where alcohol may be served. "Drinking and medical procedures don't mix," he says.

More than 1.6 million Botox procedures are performed each year, and the treatment has become the most common nonsurgical cosmetic procedure in the United States. Botox is made from a protein produced by a bacterium, *Clostridium botulinum,* and can cause drooping eyelids and asymmetry of facial features. (University of Texas Southwestern Medical Center 2002b)

Limit Your Interest in the Past

We all have a curiosity about our partner's past. We want to know about all their previous relationships and especially their previous serious relationships. But paying too much attention to this subject is dangerous. It breeds worry, comparisons, and ultimately conflict. You are not in competition with past partners—and they won't be a part of your relationship unless your feelings of jealousy or worry let them in.

SOMETIMES, THE RIGHT time is a half century in coming.

High school sweethearts Veta and Jess met in the early 1940s. War raged in Europe as Veta and Jess were finding love on the home front. Jess was off to war when he turned eighteen. When he returned home, Veta had married someone else. "I was heartbroken," Jess says.

Jess would later happily marry. For decades Jess and Veta kept up with each other through mutual friends.

Their spouses knew of the past relationship, but Jess and Veta gave their spouses no reason to be jealous. "We respected each other and each other's spouse. And that's the end of it. No what-ifs, or looking back wishing for something else," Jess says.

Within a year of each other, Jess's wife and Veta's husband died.

Several months later, Jess and Veta renewed an old friendship. Then an old romance. "I thought I was going to faint," Veta says, recalling their first kiss in five decades.

When they later married each other fifty years after their first date, there were no regrets for the circuitous path they had traveled. "We had wonderful lives separately, and we're going to have a wonderful life together now," Jess says.

More than two in five people report that jealousy over a previous relationship is a source of conflict in their current relationship. (Knox and Zusman 2001)

Don't Talk to Yourself

Answers that seem obvious to us appear that way because of our perspective—everything we know about the subject and everything we have experienced. When we communicate our ideas, though, we need to consider not just what makes sense to us, but what would make sense if we looked at the situation with a completely different background. A presentation is not the best expression of your ideas to an audience of yourself, but one of your ideas to an audience who has never seen the world through your eyes.

RETTEW ASSOCIATES, AN engineering firm in New York and Pennsylvania, surveys and plans parks, roadways, and developments.

In little more than a decade it has grown from a four-man operation to a $10-million-a-year company that has five separate divisions.

Founder George Rettew credits much of the company's success to bringing together different services under one roof: "If we can be the only firm a client has to deal with on a project, it makes life a little easier on them."

The task is not without difficulty, though, as George notes. For example, "geologists and engineers speak a different language and think differently," he points out. To overcome those problems, both for the sake of his clients and to keep his different divisions functioning well, George puts great emphasis on communication. "We need to step back and listen to each other, because there is a lot we can teach each other if we do this right," George says.

Eighty-two percent of consultants found that studying an organization's founding and long-term culture was critical to improving the consultants' ability to successfully communicate innovations. (Smith 2000)

Money Can't Buy Happiness

Money is a necessity to provide for the basics of life. But increasing sums of money do not increase our enjoyment of life, just our desire for more money.

TENNESSEE RESIDENT KIM Hunt knows what it's like to become a millionaire in an instant. A contestant on the game show *Who Wants to Be a Millionaire?*, Kim answered fourteen questions correctly and then answered the million-dollar question.

The veteran math teacher in his forties went from living on a very modest salary to having a pile of money at his disposal. Kim's first priority was to help his parents. They had provided so much for him, helping him through college, and they were now struggling with medical bills. "I was always the professional student. Always the one without money. So it was nice to be able to do something for them," Kim says.

Then he purchased some things he really wanted—a new computer and car.

But then he realized that, with few exceptions, "I'm pretty much living my old lifestyle. The money changes less than you might think. Some people ask me for money when they never did before. But I get up in the morning and I'm still the same person."

One thing that has changed, ironically, is that Kim spends more time worrying about money. "I didn't have any before and didn't think much about it. Now, I'm trying hard not do something really stupid and lose all the money. I've got it socked away in stocks and mutual funds—which sadly have actually lost some value since I bought them," Kim says.

People's rating of their own happiness does not increase as their income rises, because their appetite for products increases with their income. (Easterlin 2001)

Pay Attention to Your Dreams

Your dreams are more than a flitting source of nighttime entertainment. Pay attention to what's happening in your dreams, remember them, and write them down, because they are a central clue to what you are really feeling inside.

RIGHT AFTER FINISHING school, Monica started working as a flight attendant. She started with short flights—milk runs, they called them—back and forth between nearby cities. Over time she moved up to international flights and had her pick of European and South American destinations.

She enjoyed the work. She enjoyed the schedule. And she loved the opportunity to see the world. "For me, the job was everything I could have wanted," she says.

Monica had plans of staying in the air until she could retire. But the work started to wear on her. "When I hit fifty it really began to be physically draining. It became harder to laugh off irritating things that hadn't bothered me before," Monica says. "Like the tug-of-war with a passenger who says, 'I won't put that under my seat.' I just didn't want to deal with certain trivialities anymore."

But Monica really decided she had to make a change only when she started having a series of dreams in which she was continually isolated and scared. "There was so much negativity in my days that even when I was asleep my brain was focused on negative things," Monica says. "It was as if my body was sending me a message that it was determined I get, one way or the other."

Six months later she was working in sales. With her new job firmly on solid ground, her dreams were back to much less turbulent subjects.

People who regularly dream about negative or traumatic events are 13 percent less likely to feel satisfied with their lives. (Kroth et al. 2002)

Choose Not to Worry

Some people worry in nearly every situation. Whether things are good or bad, they worry that their situation will surely get worse. Understand that worrying is a drain on your energy and enthusiasm and that just as any situation can be used to generate worry, so too can any situation be used to generate hope.

ALTHOUGH SHE'S BARELY out of her teens, Keira Knightley has starred in a half dozen high-profile films. She faces the prospect of high expectations for her real life and her onscreen success. But she doesn't let that pressure get to her.

"With fame comes people telling me I'm a role model. That's the stupidest thing I've ever heard in my life. Don't turn someone my age into a role model, because we're going to make mistakes. How could you not? You'd be a freak if you didn't," Keira says.

Already she has faced criticism for movies that did not attract large-enough audiences. "Sometimes a movie just doesn't capture people's imagination. You never know what people are going to go for and what they aren't. It's an unforeseeable thing. I don't let that get to me—or let that affect what movies I go for. You'd be nothing but fears and worries otherwise," she says.

Keira says even from the first challenge of her life—dealing with dyslexia—she's never spent time thinking about failure: "I had to keep my grades up to be allowed to act—and I drove myself continually because that's what I wanted."

Worrying, psychologists find, is simply a matter of choice unrelated to the events in our lives. In fact, some people experience worry more than ten times as often as others, and, not surprisingly, they reduce their likelihood of happiness by 64 percent. (Tamir 2005)

A Relationship Is Built on a Foundation of Support

If you believe that your partner supports you—supports who you are, supports what you are, supports what you want and need—your relationship is built on solid ground. Give support and demand support in your relationship, and everything else will be easier and better.

THEY WERE A typical couple with young children. Since both were career minded and ambitious, they had made an agreement early in their marriage: Denise would put Jerry through school, and then he would help her while she went to school.

Everything was fine—until Denise began her studies. Jerry shirked his share of the housework and child-care duties. He began to complain about how much money her classes cost and how long she was gone.

When Denise confronted him about his behavior, Jerry said that he didn't realize that her studies would be so hard on him. Then Denise graduated and began earning more money than Jerry.

"Jerry felt like he was somehow devalued now because I was making more money. He began to see himself as a failure," says Denise.

Psychologist Warren Reed has seen this problem with increasing frequency. "Rarely do careers progress in tandem," Dr. Reed notes. "If a couple doesn't plan how they'll work through the stresses of nonparallel career paths, they will likely experience problems."

Dr. Reed advises couples that "both partners need to see the value of the support they have received from each other and that their connection to each other outweighs feelings of comparison and competition."

Researchers studying couples placed in stressful situations found that when both partners felt support from each other, they actually experienced less discomfort, with supportive couples showing 38 percent less effect of the stress on their blood pressure and heart rate. (Harris 2001)

Limit Your Piercings

The lower earlobe is the least dangerous area of the body to have pierced. Other places on the ear contain cartilage, which has a lower blood flow and will heal less quickly than the lobe.

"HALF THE BODY piercings done in this country are done by peers rather than in a professional place," says Dennis Ranalli, a dentistry professor at the University of Pittsburgh School of Dental Medicine. "Kids are doing it to each other." Indeed, you can get a piercing starter kit for $75 off the Internet; it doesn't include antiseptic, but it does have five "consent forms."

"I have one patient right now who has self-pierced her eyelids with safety pins. There's inflammation and infection there," says Dr. Ranalli, who has studied intra-oral piercing. He's familiar with a wide range of piercing-related horror stories involving Ludwig's angina (bacterial infection of the mouth tissues so severe it threatens to cut off the airway) and bacterial endocarditis (an infection of the tissues of the heart). He says there has been one report of HIV transmission by piercing, a tongue piercing resulting in a hypertensive collapse, and another resulting in cephalic tetanus.

"These aren't just localized, 'Oh, my tongue hurts' kinds of things," Dr. Ranalli says. "These could be serious, life-threatening problems. The medical profession is left treating the consequences of these things that are done for, quote, body art. So it's a problem." The irony for him, Dr. Ranalli says, is that "some of these kids won't go to the dentist because they're afraid. Meanwhile, you let somebody puncture your tongue with a large-gauge harpoon. It's strange."

The infection rate for piercings of the body other than of the lower earlobe can be as high as 50 percent. (Oregon Department of Human Services 2002)

Seek Coherence and Congruence

Individual decisions might seem ideal, but, placed in the context of a larger series of plans, those same decisions might not make any sense at all. Your goals, your plans, your daily activities and habits can't be evaluated in isolation from each other. Your purpose is not to make a series of independent decisions that by themselves make sense, but to make a series of decisions that together make sense for your life.

WHEN ISABEL AND Michael were soon to become parents, they agreed on the need for one of them to stay home with the baby. Without really discussing the situation, they both assumed Isabel would resign from her job as a nurse. They thought it was the natural thing to do: when a parent needs to stay home, it's the mother's responsibility.

While still on maternity leave, Isabel began to rethink her decision. Her income was higher than her husband's. Her medical benefits were better. What sense did it make for her to leave her job when she had the better job?

They discussed it, and although Michael was surprised at the idea, he could not argue with the financial advantages.

It took some getting used to for Michael—not earning an income, and being dependent on Isabel's salary. But the decision made sense for the family, as Michael could see. "Isabel's salary is the family's money, and our child is the best career anyone could ask for," Michael says.

Fewer than two in ten people use a decision-making strategy that encompasses how their decisions fit into all phases of their lives. Instead, people tend to rely on making the best possible decision in isolation from factors that do not seem directly related. (Ichniowski et al. 2000)

Where You Live Matters

High levels of air pollution are a significant health risk. Your decision on where to live can be as important as your decision on how to live.

FOR MORE THAN a decade, she says, local environmentalists complained that a chrome-plating operation in the San Diego area was releasing dangerous amounts of toxic chemicals. Children in the area experienced abnormally high levels of asthma and other ailments.

"Common sense tells you that if you spew a known carcinogen onto homes right next door, bad things will happen," Diane says.

Diane and others repeatedly asked for local or state officials to conduct scientific tests of the facility, but nothing happened for years. Finally, the San Diego County Air Pollution Control District arranged a monitoring program to measure airborne levels of chromium 6, a known carcinogen. Officials found dangerous amounts, exceeding all established risk models. Yet it took another monitoring effort last year by the state before the facility was finally shut down.

"Everyone had a gut feeling this was not a good place," Diane says. "We tried hard to get the science to back that feeling up, but in the absence of hard data, you have to make a judgment.

"The state spent close to a million dollars, and it took more than a decade to resolve this problem. If somebody had simply taken some precautionary measures earlier—relocating the company or buying pollution-control equipment—we could have avoided all of this and the community would have been healthier earlier."

Researchers compared people living in cities with the highest and lowest levels of average daily air pollution. Those living in the high-pollution cities were nineteen times more likely to need hospital care for respiratory conditions. (Stanford University 2002a)

Don't Let Others Set Your Goals

Too many people choose goals based on what others think. Instead, think about what you really care about, and set meaningful goals to accomplish what matters to you.

GARY LEFT THE military after twenty years of service as a marine pilot. His military friends were surprised that he would leave with the possibility of promotion dangling in front of him. How could he do this? What was wrong with him? His friends didn't quite say this to him, but that is what they wanted to know.

Gary had an answer. "Holding the highest rank has never been my dream," he told them. "It might be your dream, and that's fine, but it isn't mine."

Gary's dream was to serve his country by serving children. He offered his services to the local school district, and in a matter of a few years he was asked to run a new and rigorous high school academic program. Learning, according to Gary, is a lot like flying: "You have your hands on the controls, you have the power to excel. It's all within your hands." Teaching is, for him, a dream come true—a dream that could never have come true if Gary had worried about what other people thought he should do.

People who believe they were responsible for their decisions and their life direction are 15 percent more likely to feel satisfied. (Wiese and Freund 2005)

See the Risk in Doing Nothing

You can easily see the risk associated with big change such as applying for a new job or accepting new responsibilities. But there is a very real risk in avoiding change. If ultimately you want more, failing to take a risk can be the biggest risk of all.

WILLIAM WENT TO work each day at the General Mills plant. The work was hard and dirty, but it was steady, and William was not one to complain. Each night he came home, ate dinner, and then picked up his paintbrush.

William painted street scenes that depicted the harsh realities of city life. He painted every night for years. His works were displayed only in his closets and spare bedroom. He showed them to no one. In fact, he didn't like talking about his hobby at all if he could avoid it.

One of his friends practically begged William to enter one of his paintings in a local amateur art show.

William refused. And refused again the next year. Finally he gave in the third year, and William found himself the winner of the grand prize.

Slowly, William overcame his reluctance and allowed some of his paintings to be shown in the public library in a feature of local artwork. A dealer found the work and had to do a lot of talking but finally convinced William to let her see more. A small show and the biggest check William had ever seen soon followed.

People who are satisfied with their careers are 48 percent more comfortable accepting some risk in their job future than people who feel unfulfilled in their work. Accepting risk not only makes them feel more comfortable pursuing future opportunities, but also allows them to feel that their current position is a choice rather than a sentence. (Ingram 1998)

Your History Strengthens Your Future

Your personal history is not over. It is a part of you every day. The more you strengthen that history—by thinking about it, talking about it, writing about it—the more you will see the beauty of the life you've led and the possibilities of the life you are living.

MARY HAS LIVED through changes in everyday life she couldn't have dreamed of when she was a girl. As a child, there was no indoor plumbing in the cabin. Growing up, just trying to get some light to see at night in her family's cabin was a terrible chore. "We had oil lamps. You had to fill them, trim the wicks, and you had to keep washing the globes because they would get sooty," Mary says. Late in her teens, electricity finally came, and "all of a sudden, if you wanted light, you just turned it on."

While there was no shortage of hardships in her youth, Mary also enjoyed a close family relationship with her parents, siblings, and extended family.

It was not until she had a family of her own that Mary started writing about her experiences growing up. "My daughter said to me one time I had better put some of the stories down she was hearing from my parents, and from me, because otherwise they would be lost forever," Mary says.

Mary decided to sit down with a pen and paper and see what happened. "I was writing at first to give my children and grandchildren their history, but then I saw I was giving myself a history lesson, too. Sometimes you don't appreciate where you are until you take a good hard look at where you've been," Mary says.

People who wrote about their life histories were 11 percent more likely to feel happy with their lives and 17 percent more likely to feel optimistic about the future. (Yamada 2000)

We Look Inward
to See How People Feel About Us

People who like themselves feel liked and loved regardless of the state of their relationship and regardless of how many close friends they have. People who do not like themselves do not feel liked and loved regardless of whether they have a healthy relationship or many supportive friends.

PSYCHOLOGIST MARTIN PUGH teaches self-acceptance in counseling sessions and workshops. He says it is a trait we can't really live without.

Pugh tells the story of a patient living a passive life: "Shuffling into my office, he had all the charisma and mastery of a timid dog just in from the rain. Everything he said oozed accommodation and inferiority. 'Is it all right if I sit here?' 'I hope I'm not wasting your time with this.' 'I'm not very good at this sort of thing.'"

As Pugh delved into his patient's situation, he heard of unhappy relationships, unmet dreams and goals that had come and gone, and a daily life of worry, conflict, and endless second-guessing.

"What do I need?" the patient asked. "Medication? A support group?"

"Power," Pugh replied. "You need your power. The vital and sustaining power available that emanates from the human spirit."

Pugh told him, "Wherever you probe psychologically with someone with personal power, you hit something solid. They're always home and always grounded. Although strength of spirit is available to each of us, many never tap in and bring it to the forefront of their lives. Some simply don't believe they possess this vitality. Its presence doesn't fit with their self-image of being quiet and passive."

People with low self-esteem underestimated the degree to which other people saw them positively regardless of the strength of their relationships or the number of friends they had. (Murray, Holmes, and Griffin 2000)

Keep Variety in Mind When Exercising

Exercising for general health is best accomplished by a variety of activities. Doctors do not advise that you take up one kind of exercise to the exclusion of everything else, because doing that will put excessive strain on the muscles needed for that particular exercise while offering little reward to the muscles uninvolved in the exercise. Give yourself some variety to help keep your whole body in shape and to keep yourself interested in what you're doing.

JUSTINE'S JOB IS to promote good health habits for members of her company's health plan. When it comes to exercise, she emphasizes the value of playing the field.

"First of all, when something is fun, we are more likely to do it, more likely to stick with it. Imagine how much easier life would be if you looked forward to doing things that you now think of as a burden," she tells them.

Justine encourages people to try out as many different exercises as they can: "You will become bored with the same routine over and over again. Try a little bit of everything. Mix your regular walk with a swim, with aerobics, with a team sport. The mix will keep you interested and is better for your body.

"If time is limited, shorter workouts are better than no exercise at all, but challenge yourself to increase the duration or intensity of your exercise for one workout session each week," she says. "Don't overdo, though; and as you exercise, keep a record of your goals, and reward yourself as you improve your fitness level."

Because of the pressure placed on the small seating area, nearly 90 percent of men who exercise exclusively on bicycles have low sperm counts. (University Hospital, Innsbruck, Austria 2002)

Get Your Reality from Reality

Many of our images of relationships come from the media. The power of these media images is in the fact that we see them all the time but give them little thought. We watch a television show or a movie for entertainment and spend little time wondering about the way a person was depicted or about the stereotypes presented. Question this silly information before it becomes your basis for understanding.

"WHOEVER SAID LOVE conquers all hasn't watched television recently," says sociologist Richard Grier. "At one time, TV was filled with people in lasting, loving relationships. But on today's shows, commitment is fleeting and happy marriages are rare."

Indeed, Richard says that bailing out, or not even taking the plunge, is the primary love message of many television shows.

He points to the typical representation of a successful man on television. "Frasier Crane, first on *Cheers* and then on *Frasier,* was jilted repeatedly, then had an unhappy marriage. After a divorce, Frasier moved to Seattle, where he finds fault with every woman he meets.

"When you look around now, it's really hard to find a realistic role model," Richard says. "Most characters treat relationships as throwaway items. The few long-term couples such as on *Everybody Loves Raymond* seem not to particularly like each other." And it is not very funny to Richard that the couple with the longest-running marriage on TV is Homer and Marge Simpson.

"Almost all relationship issues are pretty darn complicated. Most of television is about sound bites, and that model for communicating is at odds with what it means to be human," he says.

Heavy television watchers were three times more likely to subscribe to stereotypes about men and women and were quicker to make assumptions about people than were those who watched less television. (Ward 2002)

It Will Get Worse Before It Gets Better

The things you most want aren't easy to get; otherwise, you would already have them. But we are faced with the daunting fact that in an effort to pursue our goals, to ultimately make our lives better, we must first endure and sacrifice. You could maximize your enjoyment of life now, which would leave you ill suited to achieve in the future, or you could maximize your effort now and create an ideal future.

"I BOUGHT A night club without really understanding what I was getting into.

"My partners were convinced it should be renovated before we opened, and suddenly my costs had tripled.

"Then we opened, and for a year, the crowds were so small I could have fit them in my living room," Dean Maples says with some exaggeration.

His experts told him it was time for a new name, a new theme, and new management. But that would mean shutting the place down, and spending even more money. "We'd already endured and sacrificed, and there was nothing to be gained by giving up now," Dean says.

Today, the Pacifica Club opens to massive crowds and generates big profits. "You can't create something like this overnight," Dean says with relief and pride.

Eighty-four percent of those in upper management report having had to deal with a "period of discomfort" in their lives. Some took career risks, worked long hours, or acquired new skills, but they saw the sacrifice as necessary to pursuing employment, promotions, and success. (Atkinson 1999)

Vote

If you had a chance to help make a crucial decision, would you want to have a voice? If you had a chance to affect the future, would you act? The process of voting—from learning about the candidates to showing up on election day—is not only a crucial civic duty; it is a means of connecting us to our community and giving us a feeling of personal responsibility.

AT A FORUM held in a South Dakota senior center, there were two things an audience of Democrats and Republicans could agree on. The first, as Fred put it, was "This campaign is a disgrace."

"Just disgusting," said Barbara. "The politicians are wasting a lot of time and money saying a lot of words, but they aren't telling us anything."

The complaints were about all the negative attacks their Senate candidates were sending out on television ads, radio ads, and mailings.

Just as upsetting as what was being said, for some, was what wasn't. "When will they have a moment to address the economy, roads, schools, the high cost of living, health care, housing? They never get to those because they are too busy calling each other names," Barbara said.

The other thing they agreed on was the importance of voting. "It's almost like they don't want us to vote. With all these negative, nonsense ads. But they can't keep me out. Even if I have to vote 'None of the above,' I'll be there," Fred said.

"I haven't missed a vote in forty-eight years," said Barbara. "It's too important to stay home. Staying home is like saying you don't care what happens to yourself or anyone else."

People who vote are 46 percent less likely to report feeling distrustful and dissatisfied with government and 8 percent more likely to report feeling satisfied with their lives. (Frey and Stutzer 2000)

Connect, See You're Capable, and Know You Count

There are basic needs we have to fit into human society. We must see that we connect to others. We must see that we are capable, capable of accomplishing important goals and making a contribution to the lives of those around us. We must see that we count—that we matter in the grand scheme of things. Each of these beliefs is central to being able to have a relationship and being able to maintain a relationship.

MOST PEOPLE WOULD be scared to take a job that required them to gain twenty pounds. Most actresses, surely, would worry that their career would be jeopardized by gaining twenty pounds in order to play a woman whose thighs wobble when she cavorts in a Playboy bunny costume. But Renée Zellweger, who did just that to play the title role in *Bridget Jones's Diary,* claims it was "a thrill. It was so much fun. I felt strange only in that I felt alien to myself sometimes.

"Weight is a very personal journey," she continues. "It's unique to each woman's experience and her own way of defining her self-image and self-worth. It's a wonderful theme in this film.

"Growing up, I never heard, 'Oh, you're so pretty.' I heard, 'Anything you want to do you can do.' I'm lucky that I didn't have those messages floating around my head from an early age of trying to match some expectations that had been projected onto me."

In seeking a relationship, she says, "it's important to know your boundaries—what you have to keep in yourself, things you must know without question. Just for purposes of survival, and to be real instead of superficial."

People who felt connected, capable, and that they counted were twice as likely to feel positive about their relationship and to feel that they were contributing to their relationship. (Conway 2000)

You Need to Know What You Are Looking For

What's the right direction for you? What career would suit your needs and abilities and help you realize your goals? What most people focus on when they ask these questions is finding out about careers, getting more information about what's out there. But before you can make sense of what's out there, you need to understand yourself. The details of a job are trivial compared to the importance of knowing who you are, what you can do, and what you want to do.

CINDY DEPPE OWNS one of the last drive-in movie theaters in Pennsylvania.

Cindy faces the same pressures that have driven almost everyone out of the drive-in business. The land is too expensive to use for movies. People don't want to sit in their cars when they can sit in air-conditioned theaters with reclining seats.

Yet, Cindy is still in the business. In fact, she says she's doing quite well.

Cindy has marketed her theater to attract not only the traditional local family-movie crowd but people who live hours away but are nostalgic for the old-time drive-in movie.

One of her friends calls her a master of marketing. Cindy says, "Well, I guess there's some truth to that, but I couldn't sell something I didn't love, and I love this place."

Those who are indecisive about their career and long-term plans are 66 percent less likely to feel that they understand their own identity. (Guerra and Braungart-Rieker 1999)

The Most Treatment Is Not the Best Treatment

Do everything you can, doctor!" It's a natural inclination, but it is not necessarily a productive one. The number of treatments you receive or the number of doctors you consult does not predict the state of your health.

A GROWING BODY of research is leading many medical experts to ask whether more is really better when it comes to health care.

Some medical specialties and geographical areas are suffering from a glut of doctors and hospitals, these experts say. Supply seems to drive demand. More hospitals in an area mean many more days spent in hospitals, with no discernible improvements in health. More medical specialists mean many more specialist visits and procedures.

"If there are twice as many physicians, patients will come in for twice as many visits," says Dr. John E. Wennberg of Dartmouth Medical School, where much of the new work is being done. "Over the course of a lifetime, what increased spending buys you is generally unpleasant interventions like intensive-care units and feeding tubes," Dr. Wennberg says.

"If you want to predict the amount of medial use, all you have to know is the medical supply," says Dr. Donald M. Berwick, president of the Institute for Healthcare Improvement, a nonprofit group in Boston. "When all is said and done," Dr. Berwick says, "the people who have been most serious about it rarely think we are underresourced. The evidence to my mind is so strong: more is not better, and it often is very, very much worse."

A study found that as much as one-third of all medical care does not improve the health of the patient. Patients receiving more care overall do not have better survival rates, nor do they have higher satisfaction with their care. (Dartmouth Medical School 2003)

Life Gets Easier

Some parts of life (mowing the lawn, moving furniture, etc.) get harder and harder as we age. But life itself tends to get easier. As we age, we tend to find deeper meaning in the things that truly matter to us. Take comfort in the thought that the most important things are getting easier, not harder.

"THE GREAT MISCONCEPTION younger people have is that older people are unhappy because of their age or spend their time wishing they were younger," says Jon Harris, a gerontologist who is old enough now to include himself among his subjects for study.

"Instead," Jon says, "age is really a blurry indicator of life quality.

"Physically, you can live your life in such a way that your body is—in effect—younger than your age. And, you can live your life in such a way that your body is older than your age. So there is no way you should feel at a particular age; it varies tremendously.

"Mentally, you can see that older folks have the capacity to demonstrate resilience and recover from difficulties in their lives that is equal to or most often exceeds that of younger people. There is an inner fortitude that comes with experience, that comes with perspective. And it is one of the talents of our more senior citizens."

Research on people over sixty revealed that six in ten showed increased optimism, less stress, and increased appreciation of others as they got older. (Kinnier et al. 2001)

Avoid the Comparison Game

When we see a friend or family member in the seemingly perfect relationship, we begin to question our own relationship. Don't let yourself play this comparison game. Your relationship must be evaluated based on your needs—not on the relative relationship success of those around you.

IT IS A relationship with a storybook start: Two friends from college promise to write to each other when the marines call him off to active duty in the Gulf War. Their letters go from friendly to intimate. A letter from a military camp in Saudi Arabia contains a marriage proposal.

More than a decade later, Tim and Karen are married with three children.

But it wasn't easy. "Any little thing could set us off," Karen agrees. "When you're young, everything is about you."

When times were at their worst, Tim fell back on his training for a business degree. "I thought about what I'd been taught in some of my business and marketing courses. It's that we have a consumer mentality. Anything can be replaced if it stops meeting our needs," Tim says. "And I was doing that to my relationship—treating it as a product and wondering if I couldn't trade it in for a better one.

"If you think about a relationship as a consumer, start comparing your spouse to others, then you've undermined what you have for what probably doesn't exist. After all, marketing isn't about making a better product, but making you dislike what you have and think what they have is better."

People who were asked first to describe an unhappy couple and then to describe their own relationship were 19 percent more likely to describe their relationship enthusiastically than were people who were first asked to describe a happy couple and then describe their own relationship. (Carsten 2001)

Cherish Animals

A nimals have so much to teach us about love. The closer we get to animals, the more joy they give us.

GINA RUNS A nursing home. She has tried all kinds of things to brighten the days for her senior citizens. What works better than anything else is dogs.

The local animal shelter brings in a vanload of small dogs every Thursday afternoon, and the seniors immediately smile. The dogs offer unconditional love, and the residents of the nursing home, who often feel isolated and withdrawn, take that love and are energized by it. Softened by the love, they give it right back to their furry friends.

"You just have to watch one of these dogs put his head under a listless hand, demanding to be petted, or rest his chin on a patient's chest and stare lovingly into their eyes, or see someone who wouldn't get out of bed offer to hold the leash and take a dog for a walk down the hall" to see how much dogs can help, according to one volunteer. "You can actually see dogs bringing people out of themselves and helping them forget their troubles. Black faces come alive, and eyes uncloud."

Interaction with animals supplies us with both immediate joy and long-term positive feelings, and contributes strongly to our happiness. Those with a loved pet are 22 percent more likely to feel satisfied with their lives. (Barofsky and Rowan 1998)

The Benefits of Alcohol
Must Be Weighed Against the Risks

Light drinking has been linked to a reduced risk of heart disease and to lower cholesterol and even to a longer overall life. However, the positive effects of alcohol are present only in a narrow range of consumption. Drinking too much overall, drinking too frequently, or drinking too much in one sitting are all habits that negate any positive effect linked to alcohol.

MARK KNOWS FIRSTHAND that alcohol can devastate a family. His daughter died after a night of binge drinking. While he has seen much progress during a career directing a dependency clinic, Mark still feels that alcoholism is the stepchild of the health-care field.

"People do not understand the magnitude of the effect of alcoholism on the criminal-justice and health-care systems," he says.

While he knows there have been health benefits associated with moderate alcohol consumption, he argues that "if alcohol were just invented today. No doctor would prescribe it. Nobody would take alcohol as a medicine with all its potential side effects."

Mark is all too familiar with the statistics on those side effects: "One-quarter of all emergency room admissions, one-third of all suicides, and more than half of all homicides and incidents of domestic violence are alcohol related. Heavy drinking contributes to illness in each of the top three causes of death—heart disease, cancer, and stroke. Almost half of all traffic fatalities are alcohol related.

"Be grateful if alcohol doesn't hurt you, but I can't see anybody counting on alcohol actually helping them."

Drinking heavily, even if infrequently, does not reduce risk of heart disease or premature death and in fact has no positive overall health effects at all. (State University of New York at Buffalo 2003a)

Own What You Do

It doesn't matter if you run a company or sort letters in the mail room; succeeding in what you do starts with taking ownership of the task. You do it; therefore, you do it well. It doesn't matter what other people are doing or what senseless roadblocks are placed in your way by dumb policies or ill-chosen leaders. What you do represents your ability, your commitment, and, ultimately, your potential to do something more.

TOM WILLIAMS BEGAN working for Apple Computer at the tender age of fourteen.

While his relationship with the company eventually soured and he was forced out before the age of twenty, he refused to look past himself as the cause.

"I can't stand people who play the victim. None of this was anybody's choice but mine. No matter how impressionable or naive I have been, it has always been my decision," Tom says.

At twenty-one, Tom works for a venture-capital firm, evaluating the feasibility of new projects. He enjoys the great personal responsibility of the position: his recommendations could gain or lose millions for the company. "It's the decisions I make, good or bad, that give me the life I lead, not the economy, not a company, not anything else," he says.

Satisfaction with work improved by 34 percent when employees felt they were individually responsible for their work output. (McCaw 1999)

Beware of Second Opinions

People tend to be far less optimistic about the relationships of others than they are about their own relationship. The people you talk to are more likely to see the negative than the positive in your relationship. When it comes to relationship decisions, you'll have to decide for yourself.

GLEN TAYLOR IS the billionaire owner of the Minnesota Timberwolves basketball team and the Taylor Corporation. Among other things, the Taylor Corporation is by far the largest wedding-invitation printer in the United States, with 50 percent of the total market.

In running his company Taylor kept a hectic business schedule, but he also had a passion for politics. "I was listening to various people who told me what was important, told me to run for governor. Said I could put my family aside for the moment," he recalls.

"My wife said she would support my decision to run. But while I was in politics, my marriage needed me full-time. My marriage was falling apart. By the time I looked up, it was too late to save it," he says.

While Taylor is disappointed that others' advice hurt his family life, he ultimately blames himself for listening to it. "I was romanced by this notion, this idea people were putting in me," he says. He calls the neglect of his marriage "the worst misstep" of his life.

"I think we all have to listen to our inner thing," Taylor says. "I pray that I don't make my decisions based on ego and don't listen to others when I should be listening to myself."

Couples were 23 percent more likely to think their relationship would continue happily into the future than were their relatives, and 17 percent more likely to think their relationship would continue happily than their friends. Not only were they more optimistic, but couples assessing their own relationship were also more accurate than their relatives or friends. (Boyer-Pennington, Pennington, and Spink 2001)

Be Realistic About Yourself

An exaggerated sense of your abilities is no more valuable to you in the long run than a stunted sense of your abilities. You do not, you should not, try to convince yourself you are Superman or Superwoman. You do yourself a disservice by trying to claim too many strengths, because such an effort will ultimately serve to undermine your confidence in the areas in which you do excel. Failure would be your kryptonite, and all your self-confidence would fade. The best self-confidence is actually based on yourself; it encompasses all your abilities, and it highlights the path to all your dreams.

BRUCE VOLUNTEERS AS a youth soccer coach on the weekends in Tampa, Florida. He enjoys coaching children, teaching them techniques of the game, fitness, and teamwork.

But what really amazes him is what happens on the sidelines.

"These parents think they are Vince Lombardi: 'Winning isn't everything, it's the only thing.' I'm focused on teaching the game, and hopefully sportsmanship, and the parents are running around like this is some cutthroat competition.

"They scream at the Refs. They scream at each other. They scream at the children. They make the kids feel like they are absolute failures anytime anything goes wrong in the game.

"It is really a devastating thing to watch—the joy of a child transformed into dejection because a parent comes to the game with the idea that their kid should be Pele instead of a seven-year-old having fun and getting some healthy exercise."

Confidence, in combination with a realistic self-appraisal, produces a 30 percent increase in life satisfaction. (Sedlacek 1999)

Adjustments Never End

L eading a satisfying life is a lot like building a sand castle. It may look great for a moment, but it will soon change, whether you want it to or not. The point, then, has to be to enjoy the process.

PATTY HAS A special perspective on the temporary nature of family life. Just three years after giving birth to their son, she lost her husband in a car accident. After raising her son on her own for more than a decade, a friend wound up in a difficult situation and asked Patty to take care of her daughter.

Through many trying times, Patty has maintained her joy in family life. "Is this always fun, always easy? No. But there are bigger things than comfort in life, and more important goals than avoiding what's important," Patty says.

Patty takes joy in watching her now teenage son and her adopted daughter make their way through school and life. "Maybe they are not as cute and cuddly as they are when they are really young, but at this age, when you talk to them, they talk back to you. And I love just that—little conversations about the world, math class, the movies.

"I have a short window—a real short window—before they go out on their own," she says. "And I'm going to teach them everything I can. And when it's time for them to go out on their own, I'm going to be sad, I'm sure, but I'm also going to look forward to enjoying them as adults."

Studies focusing on the ability of people to maintain happiness as they age reveal that an openness to change in both family life and work life is associated with a 23 percent greater likelihood of maintaining high levels of life satisfaction. (Crosnoe and Elder 2002)

Recognize the Difference Between Caution and Fear

It is easy to fear the traumatic experiences we witness on television or read about in the newspaper. But we need to recognize the difference between the legitimate dangers to our lives and the disastrous but rare events that befall people. Understand that some of the most awful and memorable tragedies you can think of are so memorable just because they are so rare.

WHEN TWO STUDENTS brought high-powered guns to Columbine High School in Colorado in April 1999, wounding and killing their fellow students and teachers, "the nation became terrified that our schools were no longer safe," says Glenn Muschert of Purdue University.

"But there is a higher probability that children will be killed in their home, die from drug abuse, get hit by lightning, or be the victim of a drunk driver than be killed in school. Our schools are safer than ever, but Columbine created fear in Americans for their children at school."

Although schools are safe compared with other settings, the danger seems bigger. "My research shows our reactions went beyond this particular event, its victims or consequences," Professor Muschert says. "Through the press reports we can see how this event affected people just as though it happened in their own neighborhood."

Professor Muschert says the fear created from Columbine and incidents like it means "youth have been increasingly thought of as being violent or as victims. This perception creates a culture of fear regardless of the reality."

The correlation between the fear of a particular kind of violent event and the actual likelihood of that event's taking place is negative. In other words, according to researchers, we tend to fear most things that are least likely to happen to us. (University of Kentucky 2002)

You'll Forget the Disagreement but Remember the Disagreeing

We remember the atmosphere, the feelings of a disagreement, long after we forget the specifics of the disagreement. Regardless of the dispute at hand, remember to always put the feelings of your partner ahead of the specific complaint, because the feelings will linger long after the complaint is solved or forgotten.

HE SELLS CARS for a living. She sells cars for a living. Adam and Sandra are both blessed with the gift of gab, with a confidence that they will get what they want when they speak to anyone. And how does that work in their relationship? "Well, you can finish each other's jokes. Because you know all the same lines," Sandra admits.

When disagreements come up, though, both see that their personalities could be a problem. "If you look at it in terms of expecting to get what you want, this could be a disaster," Adam says. "But if you look at it from the perspective that we are two people used to seeing things through somebody else's point of view, it is really a strength."

"Our trade is really about understanding," Sandra agrees. "Understanding what people are looking for and what they are all about. In our relationship, it really helps us to see what the other person is saying. We respect each other, and each other's needs, so when we disagree we really get to the heart of the matter about what is wrong, what the other person needs."

Asked to describe three recent disagreements with their partner, people had ten times as much to say about their feelings and the tone of the disagreement as they did about the topic of the disagreement. Twenty-five percent of people forgot the topic of a disagreement but could describe their feelings in the situation. (Ludwig 2000)

Don't Forget Packaging

We worry about and try to improve our performance all the time. But improving our performance doesn't do us much good if other people fail to realize what we are capable of. Don't forget that in getting what you want, appearance has to complement reality.

JAMES RODRIGUEZ RUNS a job- and life-skills program in Paterson, New Jersey called the Next Step. James works with "people who have been forgotten and cast aside." He helps get them ready to work and then helps place them.

The Next Step teaches life skills, job skills, and job-acquisition skills. "We counsel people on dressing and hygiene, and tell them the first impression that you make might be the only chance you get with an employer. It's a delicate issue, but to do justice for the person, we have to touch on it," James says.

It was ironic for James when he realized that while he spent time trying to get people to match their skills to a pleasant presentation, he didn't spend very much time at all on the presentation of the Next Step. "We worried about doing a good job, which is what we are supposed to do, of course. But we didn't worry about looking like we were doing a good job, which is what brings in more grant money and would actually allow us to help more people," he says.

Now James spends some more time on compiling statistics on the people they've helped and on producing reports on the work they do. "It's just like I tell the people I counsel: it's not enough to be right for the job; you've got to look right for the job," he says.

No other aspect of the running of small businesses is as predictive of success as the level of resources the owners dedicate to marketing. (Goldenberg and Kline 1999)

Vitamin Levels Do Not Have to Be Constant

What does a recommended daily allowance of a vitamin or mineral mean? It means what you should consume within a day. It does not mean, however, that you need one-twenty-fourth of that amount every hour, or one-fourth of that amount every six hours. Consuming the recommended daily allowance within the day is sufficient. You need not worry about timing your consumption or about using time-released vitamins.

TAKE NUTRITIONIST NANCY Reddick with you on a trip to the store and you will be in for a rude awakening when you walk down the vitamin and supplements aisle.

"It's really like the Wild West in that aisle. Anything goes. Most of these products are not regulated, and they can make any claim they want," Nancy says.

"They have products you don't need, products you don't need in that quantity, products with fancy features. With most products, the seller is not free to tell any story they want about what their product is and what it does. Supplements, on the other hand, seem to be open to the seller's creativity," she adds.

Nancy asks consumers to inform themselves before heading down the vitamin aisle alone. "If your diet does not contain sufficient vitamins and minerals, the best thing to do is change your diet," she advises. "But if you are not going to do that, choose the vitamin that meets your needs given your age, sex, and diet. Don't let yourself get distracted by the bells and whistles. Buy only what you need."

When it comes to choosing the right multivitamin, you don't have to waste extra money on time-release vitamins; regular multivitamins will do just as well. Researchers found that a constant vitamin level isn't needed by the body for the vitamins to be effective. (Tufts University 2003)

Learn to Lead Yourself

In an ideal world, you would receive the support of everyone you work with, and you would benefit from inspirational leadership from your supervisors. In a practical world, you may find yourself with a supervisor who is more a roadblock to your doing your job than a source of inspiration. As you grow more certain of your purpose and your talents, however, you will come to rely less on the attitudes and abilities of those around you and more on your own passion and ability.

AFTER TWENTY YEARS in sales, Terry Hinton laments that work "is not a career ladder, it's a career obstacle course.

"When I've had strong years, they've been written off because I've had a good territory. When I've had lean years, it's as if I'm solely responsible for the company's plight."

While the road to advancement has been blocked, salaries based on commission have provided for Terry nicely. "The reason I've been supported is, I've delivered. They've gotten hard work and profitability from me. You can't always get the respect you deserve, but you can still get the paycheck you earned," Terry says.

The productivity of employees who score high in dedication to their career is 33 percent less likely to be affected by the quality of their managers than is the productivity of low-dedication employees. Those high in dedication look for reasons to work hard instead of waiting for those reasons to be presented to them. (Pollock 1998)

Don't Let the Holidays Ruin Your Health

The holidays combine two major threats to our health in a short period of time. One is the availability of high-fat food in nearly limitless quantities. The second is the considerable stress that many of us feel because of high expectations or familial personality conflicts. Strive for a holiday that can be enjoyed, not one that is perfect. During the holiday season, drink more water and eat light snacks to limit your appetite, and don't miss a chance to take a walk.

MONICA SPENT ALMOST every Thanksgiving of her married life with her husband's side of the family in Ohio. But then the couple declined the invitation. With their son getting older, she says, they wanted to stay home and start creating their own holiday traditions. What they started, though, is a family drama with Monica as the wicked daughter-in-law.

To try to satisfy her husband's family and her own family, including her six siblings, Monica schedules as many visits as possible during the period between Thanksgiving and New Year's. "But even if we're coming for an hour, everybody feels compelled to use that time to feed you. I wouldn't want that much food in the course of a year. But you either eat or you offend, it seems."

With every passing year the pounds come, and Monica works on a strategy to accommodate everyone without having to eat her way through three states. "Of course I have to learn to say no, but it's hard to do when you are trying to please as many people as possible," she says.

The average American gains seven to ten pounds between Thanksgiving and New Year's Day. Surveys showed that anxiety levels are 55 percent greater over the holidays than at any other time of the year, which encourages what psychologists call "stress-eating." (Pennsylvania State University 2002a)

Always Think About What's Next

Of course no one knows, but there are already people more capable of dealing with the future and the changes it holds. Those people do not fear change, and they practice flexibility. Your job will not be the same in twenty years no matter what it is like today. But that doesn't mean you won't excel in the future; it just means you have to embrace innovation, because no one who fails to do so can stay on top.

BARRY AND JUDY Wirth own ProPet, an independent pet store in central Pennsylvania.

The Wirths watched as pet superstores moved into surrounding towns. These chains had massive stores, incredible selection, and the buying power to lower prices on dog food, the biggest-selling item in the pet-store business.

While Barry and Judy knew what it took to succeed with a small business that filled a unique niche, they had no idea how to face the challenge of thriving in the face of big and powerful competition.

"I looked at every aspect of what we did—and looked for things we could do better," Barry explains. Although they had long appreciated the freedom of being completely independent, the Wirths decided the future lay with a pet-supply cooperative that allowed small stores to operate with the collective buying power of hundreds of others.

Barry says the continued success of the store is dependent on one thing: "We need to keep up with the future direction of this business. If you don't change to keep up, you're going to be blindsided."

Research on employees who have experienced layoffs having nothing to do with their job performance found that flexibility—a willingness to try new tasks and learn new skills—was the single best predictor of how long people stayed unemployed. (Ingram 1998)

You Are Never Too Old to Find Love

The need for human companionship does not go away over time for men or for women. And the capacity to find joy in a relationship does not go away over time. Never give up, because you are never too old.

ROMANCE ELUDED SHIRLEY during her youth. Her marriage was a great struggle in the face of a terrible tragedy.

Her first husband broke his neck soon after their wedding, rendering her a full-time nurse for three decades, until he died. At sixty, Shirley found herself a widow, hopeful that she might discover a new love.

Undaunted by the many years since she had last gone on a date, Shirley drafted a list of requirements: He had to be under seventy-one, energetic, and spiritual. No smoking; no facial hair. He could drink socially, but not to excess. "I think the second time around you should be more fussy," she says.

Jeff was a recent widower. Friends dragged him to a seniors' outing at the local roller rink.

Shirley noticed him immediately. "Oh, I have to find out who this man is," she thought. "We breezed by each other and said hello and introduced ourselves," she recalls.

That was it—one smiling signal of interest that kept him coming back to a steady stream of senior mixers and socials.

Now they've celebrated their seventh anniversary together. They swim, walk, dance, take trips, and, of course, roller-skate. "My darling husband prepares breakfast daily and does so many thoughtful things like bringing me flowers often," Shirley says. "Loving and being loved is the greatest gift in this life. And it can happen to you anytime."

Relationship satisfaction is higher among people in their sixties than among people in their twenties. (Koehne 2000)

Stretch Out and Fly Right

Sitting cramped for a very long period of time in dry conditions can affect our circulatory system and cause potentially dangerous blood clots. Taking an airplane ride almost inevitably puts us in this situation. When flying, you can reduce your risk of circulation problems by moving around the cabin for at least five minutes every hour, massaging your legs from foot to thigh every hour, taking an aspirin before the flight, and drinking water while onboard.

AFTER MICHAEL'S FLIGHT from New York to Paris set down, he collapsed. Doctors said he had suffered a blood clot, which produced a pulmonary embolism. A clot impedes the free flow of blood, preventing tissues from getting needed oxygen and nutrients. It can become life threatening if it dislodges and travels to the pulmonary artery in the lungs. When his French doctor nonchalantly told him that such clots were common among people getting off long flights, Michael says, he was shocked.

Since then, he has been on a campaign to persuade airlines to alert passengers to the risk and advise them about what to do if they have symptoms of deep-vein thrombosis or pulmonary embolism. Michael also launched a Web site on the topic.

Michael cites statistics showing that as many as 10 percent of travelers over age fifty suffer from blood clots after long-distance flights. Other studies have found high numbers of apparent blood clots in long-distance travelers—motorists as well as fliers.

Concerned, the World Health Organization has begun studying the problem. And some international airlines are now printing warnings on tickets or showing videos on the subject before takeoff.

Researchers in Japan found that common airplane conditions reduced blood flow by 5 percent but that those effects could be reversed with proper hydration and stretching. (Saitama Medical School 2003)

Foundations Shift, but Life Stands

There will be challenges and changes, to be sure. Your resilience will see you through the good and the bad, and your capacity for making a life with happiness will persist.

HENRY WAS LIVING off his investment earnings from the stock market. He lived well and was quick to share investment advice.

Then his investments started shrinking. His broker suggested he take some of his assets out of the stock market. But Henry was convinced he had made good choices. "I said to the broker, 'I want you to stay out of my way. I do my own research. I buy when I want to buy. I sell when I want to sell,'" Henry recalls. He didn't want to sell. He waited for the market to pick up again.

But it didn't. Small losses became larger losses. And larger losses eventually swallowed his entire portfolio.

Henry sold his car. He downsized his home. And now he wears a coat inside during the winter so that he can set the thermostat lower. Henry considers his situation his own doing. "I knew I wasn't supposed to put all my eggs in one basket. But I did it anyway," he says.

Despite it all, he maintains his sense of humor. When someone says he lost his shirt in the market, Henry says, "I lost more than my shirt. I lost my socks, my shoes, my hat." But, Henry says, he learned something about himself: "I'm a heck of a lot more resilient than I thought I was."

Circumstances such as seeing one's income decline or family separate, which are related to low life satisfaction in younger people, have less effect on the long-term happiness of people in their fifties and beyond. (Diener and Suh 1998)

Closeness Cannot Be Measured on a Map

Some people live next door to family members they cannot get along with. Others live three thousand miles away from family members whom they think the world of. Regardless of the geography involved, family relationships can brighten our lives if we let them.

DONTRELLE WILLIS STORMED into major league baseball in 2003, making the All-Star game in his first season as a pitcher for the Florida Marlins.

Dontrelle credits his mother, Joyce, with his success. While his mother was a good softball player as a youngster, Dontrelle says it was her work ethic that inspired him. A welder, Joyce helped build some of California's major bridges. "There are days you don't feel like picking up that three-hundred-pound beam and you don't want to do that welding," he says. "But she had to go out and do a job to take care of me. When I get lazy or lackadaisical, I just think about her and the work she's had to do."

Dontrelle has a reputation for being one of the most down-to-earth young athletes in sports. "There's a lot of situations where a lot of people work hard and they still don't get the opportunities that they deserve," Dontrelle says.

He learned that from Joyce growing up, and he's unlikely to forget it now, because even though she lives thousands of miles away, they talk after every game Dontrelle pitches. Dontrelle says, "Just because I'm in the major leagues doesn't mean she'll stop giving advice, and it doesn't mean I'm going to stop listening to it."

In a comparison of people who considered themselves "close" to their family, researchers found there was little difference in the total amount of communication, the quality of communication, or the sharing of family information between those who lived nearby and those who relied primarily on telephone, email, and letters to communicate. (Korn 2002)

Believe You Can

We love tests and contests. We want to know who is better in everything from spelling to sprinting. We embrace the certainty that everything can be measured and that the results will tell us who can do what. Unfortunately, the most important things in life cannot be tested for. You simply have to believe in yourself—believe in the abilities, the vision, the passion, the core that brought you this far.

JEANNE KNOWS SOMETHING about living in a land of tests without really knowing your grade. Jeanne spent a career teaching drama to high school students.

"Unlike the math teacher, who not only can tell you whether you are doing well or not but can give you an exact percentage for everything you do, I can tell my students only to embrace a process," Jeanne says. After all, even the greatest performance "is not something tangible; it's the magic that happens between a performer and an audience."

The same is true for her teaching. "I have an enthusiasm for giving to my students in the classroom and in rehearsals, but if you said, 'Show it to me on a piece of paper,' I couldn't," Jeanne says.

While she wanted to become an actress, Jeanne embraced the rewards of teaching. "It wasn't the glamour and the spectacle that I had set out for, but it had it's own kind of excitement," she says.

Even without the tests and the paperwork, Jeanne won a teacher-of-the-year award. The award cited her for "bringing students into a theater experience in which they find they are capable in ways they never before imagined."

Among those soon to retire or newly retired, a belief in personal capability increases feelings of optimism for the future by 37 percent and increases feelings of happiness by 52 percent. (Efklides, Kalaitzidou, and Chankin 2003)

Hug for Health

The small acts that comfort us and show us our connection to other people are not just trivial. Not only is a hug a means to show and receive affection; it is a significant source of stress relief and comfort to our bodies.

"YOU SAY YOU'RE an M.D. prescribing hugs, and people will look at you funny," Dr. Laura Johnson says. "'Shouldn't you prescribe real medicines?' is what they're thinking.

"People imagine the body is much more like a machine than it really is. They think that fixing a person should be like fixing a machine. Just put the right parts in, and there you go. The difference is, a machine doesn't have emotions. It doesn't care how you feel about it when you put in a new part. People do care, though. You can't have a purely functional approach to healing when people are not purely functional items."

Dr. Johnson has studied the effects of personal contact, including the amount of time a family spends with a patient and the amount of time nurses spend with a patient. "The evidence is overwhelming: Everybody needs a daily dose of attention and a daily dose of touch for their emotional well-being. It is as important as diet and exercise.

"Your system is not meant to function in a cave, in isolation from everyone else. It is meant to function in a human context. Medicine has to recognize that and help people by doing so."

A brief hug with a loved one reduced the effects of stress on blood pressure and heart rate by half. (University of North Carolina 2003)

Exercise for Your Mind

Regular exercise, starting with something as easy as a daily walk, has not only physical health benefits but mental health benefits. The functioning and efficiency of the brain have been shown to improve with exercise.

THE CHILDREN START running as soon as they enter the gymnasium. They warm up, sprint, hold scooter races and more. Their physical-education teacher, Nick Cestaro, encourages them to push themselves.

"I see the energy there. That's the way to let it out," he says. The children, a group of twenty-five who attend East Syracuse Elementary School, participate in a before-school program for youths who have a hard time staying focused in class.

The program is in addition to a regular physical-education class during the school day. The before-school program aims to provide an extra release for the children, and it seems to be working. Cestaro and first-grade teacher Beth Crump say the extra activity helps pupils focus once they get in the classroom. Teachers report seeing fewer fidgeting and active behaviors and more self-control and focus.

One parent of a child in the program says it has helped improve his son's test scores by two grade levels. "Now he's coming home and doing his homework. It kicks his energy down a little bit," the father says.

"The goals are short-term. If they can get a few more hours of focus, then we've succeeded," Nick says. "They come back happy every day because it's exciting and it's fun. It's natural, and it's good for you."

Sedentary people were tested on their ability to plan, to make and remember choices, and to adapt to changing circumstances. Half were then assigned to a daily walking program, while half were not. When they were retested six months later, only the walkers showed a 25 percent improvement. (University of Illinois 2002)

You Are Complete by Yourself

A relationship is not a requirement. Your health and welfare do not require a relationship. A relationship may be a crucial part of your life and your future, but you by yourself have everything necessary to survive and thrive. Believe in yourself—regardless of your situation right at this moment—and you will be complete.

"LONELINESS IS A universal experience known to every human being on earth—single parents, teenagers, and even the happily married. Even the rich and famous," says psychologist Henry Abrams.

"Polls show that more than a third of all Americans feel lonely in an average week," he continues. "Many more of us probably have feelings of loneliness but are reluctant to admit it, feeling ashamed by our loneliness and seeing it as a sign that we are unlovable or defective instead of recognizing it as an essential part of the human condition."

But, Henry says, despite what many assume, surrounding yourself with people is not a cure: "Loneliness stems from a void within ourselves, a sense of feeling incomplete and unfulfilled even when we have many loving people in our lives. To feel complete, we need to nurture a strong connection with our inner selves. Then we can more fully connect with others and find their company rewarding."

Henry warns that feelings of loneliness often lead to behaviors, such as excessive sleeping, excessive television watching, or excessive computer use, that serve only to distract us for a moment and make us feel worse in the end. Henry's advice: "Don't take feelings of loneliness as a reason to further isolate yourself."

Researchers cannot predict feelings of loneliness based on relationship status. For example, among people currently seeking a relationship, the reported frequency of feelings of loneliness varied from always to never. (Fahrenkamp 2001)

Be Honest for Your Future

Few things are easier to lie about than the future. And few people are easier to lie to than ourselves. It is therefore not surprising that people spend lifetimes lying to themselves about where they're going and why. But lying to ourselves about our goals is like paying off a loan by taking out an even bigger loan: it makes today easier, but it makes tomorrow much more difficult.

GREG INVESTED HIS life savings in the startup costs of a handmade-soap business he wanted to start in Oregon.

There was only one problem: his handmade bars of soap turned to green mush when wet.

He'd already rented a booth in a mall and at an open market. He'd already had the labels printed. But his secret recipe for handmade soap was nothing short of a disaster.

Desperate and out of time, Greg bought soap from a wholesaler and slapped his label on it.

Greg told his customers it was handmade Oregon soap—though it was neither handmade nor from Oregon. He'd even promised in his lease to sell only his own handmade merchandise, nothing else.

Although it would have been hard for him to be caught in the act, ultimately the fraud ate him up inside. He shut down the operation and faced, among other consequences, a ban from signing future leases at the market. Still, Greg says, he's happy to be out of the deception: "If you have to lie about a fundamental aspect of your life, that builds an enormous complex in you and makes it seem like what you're doing is not even real."

People who consider their careers to have been successful are 81 percent less likely to have exaggerated their career plans when they were younger. (Ingram 1998)

Find Your Own Path

Watch cars come off the assembly line, and you will see the same functions and capabilities in model after model. People, however, are not products coming off an assembly line. Even if we emerge from the same time and place, with the same training and upbringing, our differences are present from the start and will be present forever.

Before you try to live up to someone else's expectations or to reproduce someone else's success, ask yourself whether that is what you were really made for.

EDWARD BURKHARDT ALWAYS wanted to work on the railroad.

His first job as a teenager was working on the tracks doing maintenance. After that he was a brakeman, clerk, and machinist's helper. After finishing college, he joined the front office of the Wabash Railroad. His college classmates told him he was nuts—that people didn't get engineering degrees to work for a railroad, and that the industry as a whole was dying.

After twenty years in the business, Edward put together a group to buy a regional railroad. They bought the Wisconsin Central rail lines, and began selling stock in their railroad in 1991. Even with many other railroad companies floundering, Wisconsin Central continued to produce a profit and saw its stock grow fifteen-fold over the course of the decade. Despite the old-world imagery of the railroad industry, one of the biggest investors in Wisconsin Central is Microsoft founder Bill Gates.

For Edward, success in the railroads has been a wonderful ride. "Never be afraid to pursue your dreams," he advises. "What else is there to pursue?"

Sixty-four percent of people who feel they have failed to achieve success in their lives point to a specific standard set by others that they were unable to live up to. (Arnold 1995)

Why Not Be Optimistic?

Without hope, what would you ever have tried? Nothing you've accomplished, nothing you've enjoyed would have been possible without your seeing possibilities. Seize that view to guide you to the future you desire.

CHARLES BLASBAND WANTED a job working for a dynamic employer where he had the potential to advance. Charles got a call from the head of the hospital in Citrus County, Florida, inviting him to interview for the position of the hospital's chief financial officer.

When he drove to the hospital, he thought he must have had the address wrong. He was staring at an unassuming one-story building that hardly resembled any hospital he'd ever seen. After a tour of the facility, the hospital's CEO took Charles out for a drive in the surrounding area. Charles thought he was wasting his time.

Driving down through rural farmland, the CEO told Charles that he thought the hospital had potential, that Charles had potential, and that Charles could be running the hospital before long. His skepticism, Charles says, melted away at the sound of those "magic words." Sure enough, six years later Charles was promoted to CEO.

As Charles's responsibilities grew, so too did the hospital. His leadership brought an expanded emergency room, new operating rooms, and a new building for physicians. He tripled the number of beds and created a heart-care facility offering the only open-heart procedures anywhere in the region. The typical hospital executive stays on the job for about five years. More than twenty-five years later, Charles is still running Citrus County Hospital. "I just thought this was a bump in the road," he says. "But then I thought it could be something more."

People with a tendency to see things optimistically were 29 percent more likely to feel a sense of well-being. (Lounsbury et al. 2003)

Your Life Has Purpose and Meaning

You are not here just to fill space or to be a background character in someone else's life story. Consider this: nothing would be the same if you did not exist. Every place you have ever been and everyone you have ever spoken to would be different without you. We are all connected, and we are all affected by the decisions and even the existence of those around us.

ACTOR JEFF DANIELS has appeared in movies that have won huge audiences (*Speed* and *Dumb and Dumber*) and in movies that have won widespread acclaim (*Terms of Endearment*). But he's never lost his love of the theater.

"I started on Off Broadway, and I really never wanted to leave. In movies, it's too easy to be totally disconnected from the audience," Jeff says.

Even after he gave in to the lure of movies, his heart remained in the theater. So much so that he founded the Purple Rose Theater Company in his Chelsea, Michigan, hometown. The theater, named after the Woody Allen movie he appeared in, attracts more than forty thousand people per year to a wide array of shows, including some Jeff has written.

"It's out in the middle of nowhere, it has absolutely no reason to succeed whatsoever, and it's doing really well," Jeff says. "Just to see people in the building is a thrill for me. This is their Broadway, and they're getting the connection that only theater can give you in a place where they really don't know what theater is. But because of the Purple Rose, now they do."

Studies find that one of the best predictors of happiness is whether a person considers his or her life to have a purpose. Without a clearly defined purpose, seven in ten individuals feel unsettled about their lives; with a purpose, almost seven in ten feel satisfied. (Steger et al. 2006)

Can I Do It? Ask Yourself

You cannot do more than you think you can do. But you can do what you think you can do.

IN EBONY'S STORY, the turtle with attention deficit disorder beats a rabbit at a spelling bee because he learns to believe in himself and to work at his own pace. Ebony based the story on her own life of overcoming obstacles and succeeding.

Today, Ebony has dedicated herself to learning how to be the best parent she can be. She recently took part in the Hartford, Connecticut, school district's Parent Power Institute.

The program teaches parents storytelling, literacy, and computer skills with the goal of making them more involved in the education of their children. Like Ebony, many participants say they learn more than just computers and communications during the program, describing how they have gained new confidence about speaking out and setting goals for themselves.

The program emphasizes the importance of reading to your children, which Ebony has taken to heart. "If you read to your child, you're teaching them not only to read, but also bonding," she says. "And with the right story you can show them that they can do anything, be anything they want to be. It's that belief that's at the start of anyone doing anything, including being a good parent."

Ebony had no problem deciding what to read next to her child. "It's a story about a turtle and a spelling bee," she says.

Feeling personally capable reduces by 28 percent the likelihood that a person will feel overwhelmed by work and family. (Erdwins et al. 2001)

Pets Are Healthy

There are few things in life that are inherently sources of calm and good cheer. One of those is a family pet. Pets give us unconditional love and a steady, positive form of responsibility, and they offer us comfort regardless of what else might be going on in our lives. As a result, we are actually healthier when we live our lives with pets.

WENDY HAS SHARED her life with dogs for as long as she can remember. "When you come home from work after a long, hard day, who is the first family member to greet you at the door? In my house that would be Arthur, our Irish setter. He jumps up and down on his big feet and spins in circles. He barks. He looks at us with loving eyes that indicate that by merely walking through the front door, we have made him the happiest dog in the world," Wendy says.

While she thought of her dog as a source of love, she never thought of him as a source of health. Then a friend of hers was "prescribed" a dog as part of her treatment for cancer.

Wendy read up on the subjects of pets and health. "Ninety-seven percent of pet owners in a survey reported that their pet makes them smile at least once a day. Seventy-six percent believe their pet eases their stress level. People who live with dogs even go to the doctor less often than people who do not," Wendy says.

While she always loved and appreciated her Irish setter, it's hard for her not to feel even more indebted to him now. "We used to think of a him as a watchdog for the house, but he's also a watchdog for our health," Wendy says.

Pet owners are 15 percent less likely to suffer from high blood pressure than non–pet owners. (State University of New York at Buffalo 2003b)

Have Faith, but Don't Forget Reality

Faith that things will work out should not lead us to think that every day will be perfect. Believe in the future, but believe, too, in the work it will take to make that future what you want it to be.

PROFESSIONAL GOLFER JIM Furyk volunteers from time to time to give golf lessons to youth groups. He often sees a youngster pick up a golf club for the first time and take a mighty swing at a ball. "They try a home-run swing, to hit it as far and as hard as they possibly can," Jim says. And what happens? The ball usually goes a little left, a little right, but not very far at all.

"It doesn't make sense, does it?" he asks. "You swing with control, and the ball goes farther than if you swing with your all. But, golf doesn't make sense."

Jim has honed his skills with literally hundreds of thousands of practice swings. Like any professional, "I've learned what I can and can't do," he says. "And I've learned that you had better focus your attention on what you can do or you're not going to last very long."

But Jim, who won the U.S. Open championship in 2003, says he appreciates the golden rule of golf: "As Bobby Jones said, 'Golf is a game of luck. And the more I practice, the luckier I get.'"

Although their expectations are statistically impossible, studies show that more than seven out of ten Americans expect to have an above-average income in the future. (Chambers and Windschitl 2004)

Be Careful What You Ask For

The ads are everywhere on television and in newspapers and magazines. "Ask your doctor" about a new medicine, they tell us. When people ask about a medication, more often than not they get prescribed that very medication. It is almost making you the doctor, diagnosing your own ailments and thinking up your own treatment plans. Be careful when making suggestions to your doctor, and instead of asking about specific drugs, consider asking about your condition and seeing whether the doctor thinks medication is needed.

TELEVISION AND PRINT advertising for prescription medicines that is aimed directly at consumers is soaring in the United States. So is the average American's spending on drugs.

Critics see a connection. They say ads are persuading Americans to buy drugs they don't need and are driving up the costs of an overburdened health-care system. Nancy Chockley, president of the National Institute for Health Care Management, reports that the fifty most heavily advertised drugs accounted for almost half of the $21 billion increase in drug sales in the United States between 1999 and 2000. The ninety-eight hundred other drugs accounted for the other half.

"It's very hard for physicians to say no to these drugs," Nancy says. "You want that drug, your doctor writes a prescription in two minutes, and you walk away happy. If a doctor tells a patient he doesn't need it, the patient thinks, 'Gosh, he doesn't think I'm in pain.' It takes a half hour for the doctor to explain, and the patient leaves unhappy." Chockley notes that most doctors admit that, because of patient requests, they have prescribed drugs they would not ordinarily recommend.

When patients ask their doctors about a drug they've seen advertised, 69 percent of the time the doctor winds up prescribing the advertised medicine to the patient. (Food and Drug Administration 2002)

Take Action

Sharks have to keep moving forward to live. People need to keep moving forward in order for their dreams to live. You do not need to do everything today, but you do need to do something every day.

MICHAEL FRANKLIN HELPS make sure everything we order gets to our doors on time. He is a vice president for one of America's largest shipping services.

When the company brought in a consulting firm to assess the workplace climate and the leadership skills of executives, many were skeptical or even offended.

But Michael says he saw this as an opportunity: "I am past the point of being able to be embarrassed, but if there's something they could point out or teach me that's going to make me a better manager, or put me in a better position to advance, then I want to know about it."

The profile that emerged from the consultants noted positively his energy, drive, persistence, and hustle, but suggested he could improve his ability to communicate and relate to other employees.

Michael took the report and started scheduling meetings with people above and below him in the company. "I'm very plan focused, so I took what they had to say and I immediately tried to put it to use. I think it's made me better at my job already," Michael says.

Those who do not feel they are taking steps toward their goals are five times more likely to give up and three times less likely to feel satisfied with their lives. (Elliott 1999)

Health Is About Life

We see stories on the news about the latest pill, the latest treatment, the latest and most expensive remedy for whatever ails us. What we don't see touted is that the route to a healthy life is not found in doctors' offices or hospitals. It is found in our homes and in our lives. Enjoying your life and the people around you will contribute to your health and reduce the effects of aging.

FOR BETH, TWENTY years of dieting seemed nearly at an end. She saw an ad for a prescription weight-loss drug that blocks fat absorption in the digestive system. She discussed it with her family doctor, who prescribed a month's supply.

Soon Beth learned the drug had an unpleasant side effect: sudden-onset diarrhea.

The drug is supposed to encourage dieters to stick to a low-fat diet because it makes excess fat in food leave the body through bowel movements. But even though Beth wasn't eating a high-fat diet, half an hour after eating, "you'd have to be close to a bathroom," she says.

The more she thought about it, though, the more she came to have doubts about the whole concept. "You can't be on a drug forever," she says. "The weight will come back. You go back to old habits that put on the weight in the first place. If you don't change your life, there's simply no point to quick fixes." After going off the medication, Beth focused on reducing her daily calorie intake and walking every day.

She says she is relieved to be focusing on a healthy lifestyle instead of just on losing pounds. "I do feel better about myself, and I'm not always looking out for the nearest bathroom," Beth says.

People who described their home lives as satisfying were 24 percent more likely to live beyond normal life expectancy. (University of California, Los Angeles 2002)

The Search for Perfection Is Endless

There is a difference between looking for something that is healthy and satisfying and looking for something that is perfect. The difference is that healthy and satisfying exist; perfect doesn't. Seek fulfillment, and you will find it; seek utopia, and you will be looking forever.

CHRISTINE, A COMPUTER programmer in Florida, was living with her boyfriend but questioning her decisions. "I was learning things. I don't think you'll ever really know a person unless you really have to share everything with them," she says. But she wasn't sure about which direction to take. "I mean, on the one hand, it was like, 'Oh my God, his feet smell!' and on the other hand, he seems to be a nice guy. But I didn't know if this is what I wanted forever," she says.

They lived together for a year. They seemed to be happy. Then they happened to see the film *Indecent Proposal* on cable one night. After the movie, she asked him if he'd trade her in for $1 million. He said, "Not for $1 million, not for $10 million."

"And I thought that was sweet. And I realized I just liked and loved him so much, I wanted to spend my life with him," she says. "I just knew he was the guy for me. I just followed my heart." They got married. They're still happy.

"Day to day, it's all about compromise," she says. "'It's about giving in and saying you're sorry or dumb, as the case may be, and being sometimes brutally honest. Because love isn't about two puzzle pieces that fit together perfectly, but two people with similarities and differences, and strengths and weaknesses."

People high in perfectionism—who have an overwhelming belief in their own correctness and a desire to find a partner with similar traits—are 33 percent less likely to describe their relationship status as satisfying. (Flett et al. 2002)

Win Your Own Respect First

You can't make your success contingent on someone else's reaction. Competing to impress your parents, your spouse, your co-workers, or anybody else will ultimately not be fulfilling. You can't conform to their every hope and expectation, and you will experience great frustration when your accomplishments prove insufficient to gain their approval. If you start with a respect for what you can do that depends on no one else, you will have a much easier time tolerating those for whom nothing is enough.

"IT'S A VICIOUS cycle," reports educator Sally Tucci. Every day she watched inner-city children compete with each other to see who can learn less.

"Somewhere along the way they failed, and they became afraid to try," she says. "Since they're unwilling to try, they have to make trying the failure and failing the success. Students mock anyone who answers a question, who carries their books home at night, who asks a question. The lesson is that if you want to fit in, you better not learn."

Sally says she tries to break down these attitudes every day: "I say if your friends tell you up is down and down is up, are you going to listen? You have a chance in this life to do something, but not if you spend your time listening to someone who wants you to do the opposite of the right thing."

Sally attacks the fear as the first step toward building self-confidence. "You have to think about the things you can do instead of the things you can't do—and you'll be amazed at how many things you can do."

Researchers find that an optimistic personal outlook is more than just seeing the bright side of things. Believing in yourself actually produces better health as well as increases in motivation and achievement for six in ten people. (Schulman 1999)

Think As If Others Can Read Your Mind

A number of science-fiction movies have considered the idea of the havoc that would be wrought if someone could read minds, could hear other people's private thoughts. While no one can do that, people do accurately perceive others' level of job satisfaction. Your co-workers, your customers, your family—they all have a good understanding, even if you haven't directly said anything, of how satisfied and committed you are to your job. Realize that in your tone, demeanor, and body language you are communicating thoughts you have about your job.

MICHAEL PHIPPEN RUNS a temporary staffing agency in Florida called Staff Leasing.

When he took the top job in the company, he spent nearly all his time talking with sales associates. "Nothing begins until you sell something, and they're the first line of folks who know what our customers want, what our customers need, and what we're delivering," Michael says.

He learned that there was a disconnection between the different groups in the company. Sales and operations were not on the same page, and the customers were lost in the process.

Michael says he set out to bring everybody together in everything they do: "My success has been in taking disparate areas of the organization with different focuses and bringing them together, to see the common needs of the company, and ultimately to create a winning scenario based on all of the pieces of the puzzle, not just their focus.

"Once we did that, we began to win those customers back who saw this is really one organization with one purpose."

Co-workers and customers asked to rate the job satisfaction of retail-store employees were three times as accurate as random chance. Customers were 70 percent more likely to continue to do business in a store if they found the employees satisfied with their jobs. (Hagan 1999)

Don't Drown Yourself in Water

Water gets a lot of attention in health circles, and rightfully so. It is the healthiest drink and should be a significant part of your liquid intake. But there is no reason to consume water as if you're in a water-drinking competition. The positive effects of regularly drinking water do not translate into supereffects if you drink even more water. You do not need to force yourself to drink water.

DR. HEINZ VALTIN of the Dartmouth Medical School has studied water and its effects. He says there is simply no evidence to back the popular notion that people should drink eight glasses of water a day.

Dr. Valtin, a kidney specialist, sought to find the origin of this notion and to examine the scientific evidence for it. He observes that we see the exhortation everywhere: from health writers, nutritionists, even physicians. But Dr. Valtin finds it "difficult to believe that evolution left us with a chronic water deficit that needs to be compensated for by forcing a high fluid intake."

Dr. Valtin thinks the notion may have started when the Food and Nutrition Board of the National Research Council recommended approximately "1 milliliter of water for each calorie of food," which would amount to roughly two to two and a half quarts per day. Although in its next sentence the board stated that "most of this quantity is contained in prepared foods," that last sentence may have been missed, so that the recommendation was erroneously interpreted as how much water a person should drink each day.

Despite the dearth of compelling evidence, then, what's the harm? "The fact is that, potentially, there is harm even in water. Too much can overload the kidneys," explains Dr. Valtin.

Typical foods consumed on a daily basis provide as much as 100 percent of the water consumption experts advise. (Pennsylvania State University 2002c)

Relationships Are Like Modern Art

While there are many things that successful relationships have in common, much of the time a person's reaction to the state of their relationship is purely personal and unrelated to specific events or factors. In other words, what you see in the relationship depends on how you look at it and what you are looking for.

"YOU CAN'T HAVE what someone else has. You just can't," says Elaine, a nurse. Unhappily married in her twenties, and happily married in her forties, Elaine has learned something about perspective.

"First of all, to literally have what someone else has, you'd have to take it away from them. Second, even if you did that, you still wouldn't have what they have, because part of what they have is themselves," Elaine says.

"I wish that I had known somebody who I could have talked to before I got married," she says. "I was completely unprepared to create something. I thought of marriage almost like you would think of buying a house. You pick out one you like, one something like a friend has. Then you buy it, and it's yours.

"It doesn't work that way, of course. Marriage is more like you buy the materials, and now you have to figure out how to use them, how to build something with them.

"What I learned through experience is that I had to figure out what I wanted for me, and not for anybody else. You have to take the burden off yourself of trying to re-create anything. Instead, you will be better off creating your own unique relationship for you and your partner."

Studies of happily married couples found that in more than half of all couples, idiosyncratic factors, aspects that varied from marriage to marriage, were important in understanding marital satisfaction. (Bachand and Caron 2001)

Keep Your Goals Where You Can See Them

Your goals should be an ever-present part of your life, offering you direction and encouragement. Don't come up with a list of goals, hide them away somewhere, and check back forty years later to see if you reached them. Create them, use them, follow them, update them, live by them.

CONNIE IS A student counselor in Milwaukee. She works with high school students to get them thinking about their futures and to begin considering possible careers.

"The biggest thing is to get students started," Connie says. "So many of them have no concept of what they might want to do, which means they never consider the things they will have to do to become what they want to be.

"We start talking with them, seriously, to give them a reality check, so that they can start formulating their goals.

"Career planning is a lifelong process, but the sooner we start, the better chance we have of making decisions that will benefit us down the line," Connie explains. "Once students have a goal, they get not only a sense of direction for what they're doing, but also a sense of purpose."

Successful people spend at least fifteen minutes every day thinking about what they are doing and can do to improve their lives. (Sigmund 1999)

Make Health a Convenience

It sounds strange to imagine considering convenience when thinking about health. But people tend to factor in all the costs to themselves, whether in time or money, when they are making their health decisions. In decisions ranging from your daily schedule to choosing a place to live, make it easy for health to fit into all your plans.

DENIS IS A navy veteran living on the west coast of Florida. When the Veterans Administration combined its health facilities with its benefits office in Bay Pines, Florida, he saw the effects immediately.

Denis was a patient in the V.A. medical center and a client in the career-counseling center of the benefits office. "When they were two separate operations, fifty miles apart, you would have to make a choice between going to one or going to the other," Denis says. "Now they are in the same place, so the checkup I might have skipped because it was too far out of my way is now next door to where I was going anyway.

"Before, some people felt like it was a conspiracy, like they were trying to make it tough for us to use these services," Denis says. "This kind of disproves that. It's going to be good for a lot of veterans."

The department also reorganized the way it responds to inquiries, so veterans can immediately talk with someone familiar with their cases rather than getting passed from person to person. "We are trying to make things as convenient as possible," V.A. spokeswoman Margaret Macklin says, "because we've found our services are more valuable when they are easy to access."

A study found that people who lived close to a hospital were 15 percent more likely to choose therapies their doctors recommended over more convenient therapies that required fewer hospital visits. (Duke University 2003)

Don't Settle

People don't buy houses or cars if they're not sure about everything. These decisions are too important to rush into that kind of commitment. But how many of us toil in jobs that we don't think are right for us. You will spend more time between the ages of twenty-five and sixty-five working than you will doing anything other than sleeping. Not only will your job define possibilities for your future; it may come to define you. Never stop thinking about what you need to do to love what you do.

WILLIAM RASPBERRY IS a Pulitzer Prize–winning columnist for the *Washington Post*. He loves his job and wishes more people loved theirs.

"You need to love what you do," William says. "Love the hell out of it. Don't settle for just liking your career, for becoming a data processor or school principal or Toyota saleswoman because 'The paycheck's decent, and hey, it's a job.'"

He has a simple test for figuring out if you're in the right line of work: "Imagine the job you have right now paid you the least amount of money you could possibly live on. Would you still want the job? If not, you're not in the right line of work."

Even though they may not want to, people tend to take their jobs home with them at the end of the day. Low levels of career interest are associated with low enjoyment of life overall and even greater dissatisfaction with family life. (O'Brien, Martinez-Pons, and Kopala 1999)

People Who Have It Right Work Harder to Make It Better

You might think that people should work hard to get something right, and that once they do, their efforts would decrease. In truth, people who work hard to get something right tend to keep working hard to get it even better.

FOR KAREN ROGERS, the revelation occurred as she implemented an incentive pay program at the property-management firm she runs. An off-par year for the company forced her to seek alternatives to across-the-board salary increases. Instead, she devised an incentive plan that would be based on a combination of overall profit and personal productivity.

To see what effect the incentives had, she carefully charted the output of every employee. "The investment in time was immense, which is the great hidden cost of incentive plans," she says.

When she compared productivity before and after the plan was introduced, she found that nearly one-third of her employees did not increase their output. When she broke the results down further, it became clear that the employees who had not improved were generally the most productive to begin with.

Two years later, when Karen scrapped the incentive plan, she dug out the numbers again. Sure enough, there was a group of workers whose productivity had not meaningfully changed. And it was the same group.

Karen says of what she learned from the experience: "The definition of a good employee is someone who already does what you think you might need an incentive plan to get other people to do."

Managers of production facilities who are meeting their quality targets actually invest 20 percent more time in improving their practices than managers of facilities that are falling short of their goals. In other words, the better work harder to get even better. (Coulthard 1998)

What Is the Point?

I f you could pick one thing you most wanted out of your job and your life, what would it be? While many of us chase money, prestige, and recognition, the single most important thing you can achieve is meaning. Having a purpose in everything you do makes every day valuable and every outcome, good or bad, worthwhile.

BARBARA MILLER IS a consultant who studies the workplace and the quality of workers' lives for high-tech companies.

Barbara explains that "the global marketplace is requiring organizations to be open around the clock now, and that is changing both the work and the lives of high-tech employees."

Barbara warns companies that they cannot overlook the strain they place on families when the workday expands or becomes limitless.

She reports that many companies talk about the work/life balance but then don't practice it: "Just putting in work/life programs isn't going to help people have work/life harmony. We've really got to take a look at the way organizations are structured and change our workplaces accordingly."

Barbara found one organization in which all its engineers were on call every weekend in case of a client emergency. "Anyone could be called away from their families at any time," she says. "They could never really relax, because they didn't know if they were really off or not. Turnover was very high, because many of these people questioned why they would want a job that prevented them from having a life."

Ultimately, Barbara's recommendations were followed and a new policy was created where weekend shifts were scheduled and staffed voluntarily by workers who received weekdays off in return.

Feeling there is meaning in your life is eight times more likely to produce satisfaction than is a high income. (King and Napa 1998)

It's Not Easy, Even If It Looks It

We all know someone who seems to lead the perfect life, with the perfect love. The truth of the matter is that relationships are work for everyone. There are no perfect love stories. There are many stories of dedication, devotion, and a willingness to work through the hard times—but everyone struggles through difficulties in finding or maintaining their relationships.

WHEN JOE AND Maria and their three sons moved to Ohio, their new neighbors thought a perfect family had moved in. But Joe and Maria knew their ten-year marriage was on shaky ground.

"From every appearance, we looked like we had it all together," says Maria. "We went to church. We got along with each other in public. We were involved with our kids' lives. But Joe and I were struggling to maintain the image. We spent nearly all our time blaming each other for just about everything.

"It was as if divorce was calling ahead to say we should anticipate a visit," Maria says. "And in my heart I knew it wasn't just Joe's fault. I was equally to blame. But I had trouble keeping that idea in the middle of an argument."

Both Joe and Maria sought counseling and have worked hard to adopt a new approach to each other and to their lives. "Keeping our marriage on a positive track is not a piece of cake," Joe admits. "But it's amazing how much easier it is when you remove the land mines from self-centered lives. Maria and I are learning to keep better standards with each other."

Researchers found that more than nine in ten people could name someone they considered to be an ideal couple and that most felt disappointed that they could not match the couple's relationship success. (Taylor 2001)

Hope Springs Internal

We look around at the economy, at what's going on around us, and we size up our prospects. Will we make it? We consider every external factor we can find. But the best information you have is not national economic reports or even the company newsletter. It is your own approach, and it starts with two simple beliefs: you can get the job done, and you can show others that you can get the job done.

JAMES BLACK WORKED in a department store helping decide which clothes the store would sell. But he was convinced he could make better clothes than what the store was selling and that he could make more money doing it.

His co-workers told him it was a long shot and that he should know better than to try.

James was not discouraged, however, and he launched jimmy?WEAR in 1995. He has worked long hours, and his clothes have steadily gained a foothold in stores across the country.

James has one strategy for persevering in the fashion industry, which revolves around intense competition and constant rejection: "No matter what you are trying for, you can't let a 'no' mean 'no.'"

Nine in ten people who believe they will one day realize their career goals have strong feelings of competence and assertiveness. (Velting 1999)

Completely Healthy Is Rare

An interest in health is a very useful thing. An obsession with health is, however, a dangerous thing. Most people have some health concerns at any given moment of their lives. Understand that this is normal and that your concern should be to minimize health problems, not eliminate them.

CORBIN LACINA OF the Minnesota Vikings tells his teammates to cheer up when they step onto the field for the first day of training camp, which is a monthlong series of practices preceding the regular season. "Just remember how you feel right now. Because it's the best you're going to feel for six months."

Players agree that the toughest part of their job is the day after a game. "You wake up Monday morning, and the first step out of the bed is one of the most painful things in the world. I've had times when I literally think, 'How do I do this?'" teammate Byron Chamberlain says.

"They say a game is like having twenty or thirty car crashes or something like that," Vikings receiver Chris Walsh says.

The majority of the Vikings don't get badly injured, however. Most won't be listed on the team's weekly injury report. But that doesn't mean they're not practicing and playing with considerable discomfort.

"You become desensitized to it. You just have to realize that's just the way you feel all the time during the season," Corbin adds. But there is one sure way to ease everybody's pain. And that's winning. "Of course," Byron says, "everything is a little better when you win. And everything hurts a little worse when you lose."

Researchers found that less than 19 percent of Americans could be classified as completely healthy, with high levels of physical and mental health and low levels of illness, at any given moment. (Emory University 2002a)

We Seek Warmth

You don't have to be perfect. You don't have to be exciting. You don't have to be funny. You don't have to be wise. The most important thing you can offer your loved ones is something that is within us all: genuine concern.

CONGRESSMAN MARK FOLEY of Florida knows what it's like to have dedicated parents. The youngest of five children, Mark says his parents were always eager to show their love and devotion.

When Mark decided, soon after graduating from high school, that he wanted to open a restaurant in his hometown, his father helped him remodel the space while his mother helped out with the cooking. After serving on the local town council and then in the state legislature, Mark was elected to Congress. His parents came to Washington to see him sworn in, and when they discovered that the office space he'd been assigned was a dusty corner of what had been the House Office Building attic, his mother started cleaning the windows and his father polished the furniture.

After he was reelected to Congress four times, Mark decided the time was right to run for the U.S. Senate. Mark crisscrossed the state of Florida speaking to political groups and asking for support. He was among the leading candidates when he got the news that his father had cancer and the doctors were concerned it was spreading. Mark was stunned and soon gave up his senate campaign. Mark explained at the time that he needed "to spend as much time with my parents as I can. It was the most mature decision of my life: to show them the love they have always shown me."

Studies of adult children find that nine out of ten feel closest to the family member who showed them the most warmth and sensitivity. (McCarter 2000)

Don't Run in the Wrong Direction Just Because You're Near the Finish Line

How many times do you finish things even when you wish you hadn't started? We keep going because we've already started, not because it makes any sense to continue what we're doing. Be prepared to stop—not based on what you've already invested, but based on how much you stand to gain by continuing.

BRAD RUNS A high-tech security firm and sees the inside and decision-making process of all kinds of companies.

"The most amazing part of this business," Brad says, "is the number of times you'll hear that a business is concerned that their security is inadequate but that they can't make a change right now because they're already paying for another system."

"Well, if you're already paying for another system that doesn't work, you're not really paying for security.

"I really question when management teams refuse to make a change, even after they acknowledge the need for it, because they don't want to look bad for having made the wrong decision the first time, or they don't want to waste the money paying twice for something.

"When I hear that, I wonder if they can ever adapt to their environment, or if they will go down in flames because they had something written down that was the plan no matter what."

In experimental settings, people rate the feasibility of continuing the development of a new product more strongly based on its nearness to completion than on the likelihood of the product's producing a profit. (Boehne and Pease 2000)

Do It Now

The most vital belief you need in order to live your life is that actions matter. Actions are called for. Actions are rewarded. Take action now. There's no reason you shouldn't, and many reasons you should.

"I'M AN ACTION guy. I've got to be doing something," Dan says.

Dan spent a career fighting fires in upstate New York. He says he chose the work because he wanted to do something: "The fire department looked like it would be pretty exciting. Whenever I saw a fire truck race by with those guys hanging off the back, I said, 'That looks like something that would hold my attention.'"

When he reached his midfifties, he had already surpassed the typical retirement age in his department. So Dan retired, at least in theory.

Before his papers were even complete, though, Dan found work with the Federal Emergency Management Agency.

"Retirement from the fire department doesn't make me slow down," he says. "It's an opportunity to speed up."

FEMA has sent him to Puerto Rico, Louisiana, Kentucky, New Jersey, New York City, and Iowa after hurricanes, floods, tornadoes, and other disasters, and Dan helps people put their lives back together.

"It's an exciting job," Dan says. "They call me and they say, 'Get your gear.' Then you get on the plane and go.

"In this job, you get to see parts of this country you don't normally see, and you don't do it as a tourist," Dan says. "You go to where something's happening. You help people. For a moment, you become part of the community." And then, a few weeks later, "you do it again someplace else."

The feeling that actions taken would be unlikely to produce results produced feelings of apathy and boredom in 74 percent of people studied. (Bargdill 1998)

Happiness Is Not an Accident

We have strategies for everything in our lives—from work, to games, to how to get home from town two minutes faster. But some of the most important parts of life, like our happiness, we leave to chance. Happiness is not like height; you don't just get a certain amount and then have to live with it. Happiness can be improved—if you know what you are doing and what you are not doing, and care to change.

IT STARTED WITH a request from a neighbor. He had played the part of Santa Claus, creating a tradition in the neighborhood. One year he had a cold and wondered if Patrick could take over for him that day.

Patrick donned the suit and passed out candy canes and good wishes to all the neighborhood children. "When I put on the suit, I actually felt like Santa Claus," Patrick says.

When the old Santa saw how much Patrick enjoyed the job, he told him he would be happy to let him take over. Patrick saw the potential for sharing some joy with others and expanded his duties from his neighborhood to visits to area hospitals. "Sick children would light up when they saw me," Patrick says.

Over the years the Santa suit wore out and Patrick upgraded to a top-of-the-line model. "The kind they use at the really good malls," he explains.

Patrick has been Santa so long now that he's beginning to see the children of the children he saw as Santa when he first started out. But Patrick has no plans to find a new man for the suit. "Santa never retires," he says.

Researchers found that the majority of subjects studied were not able to identify anything they had done recently to try to increase their happiness or life satisfaction. (Frijters 2000)

Master Your Fears

All social interactions require you to reveal something of yourself. For many people, this process is nerve-racking because we fear that what we say and do won't be good enough and will be cause for rejection. People overcome these fears in one of two ways. Either they come to believe that everything they say and do will be adored, or they let themselves not care about winning everyone else's approval every moment of the day. Abandon the fear of negative reaction and the need to edit yourself moment by moment—because those who react positively to the real you are the people whose company you should seek.

"HOLIDAYS BRING OUT pain for many. People tend to hold unrealistic expectations of what the holidays will bring—lingering kisses under the mistletoe and declarations of love rivaling Romeo and Juliet," says Professor Susan Brown.

"Commitment seekers often use the holidays to mark the progress of their relationship and mistakenly assume that 'if we're together for the holidays, we're together forever,'" Professor Brown says. "They tend to analyze every detail and judge the relationship by what happens, fearing that if their expectations are not met the relationship is doomed."

But Professor Brown warns that "in this situation, people sometimes sabotage their relationships, or their chances to start a relationship, because it's the only way they can breathe. They will pick a flaw, change plans, become difficult or argumentative. They seize opportunities to create distance." Professor Brown thinks "feelings of fear and doubt should be acknowledged but not acted upon. Give yourself permission to feel uncomfortable and not be perfect."

Eight in ten people who had recently started a relationship were affected by feelings of social anxiety similar to those felt by someone meeting a group of strangers or starting a new job. (LeSure-Lester 2001)

Nice People Don't Finish Last

It's a popular notion to think that nice people are overlooked while other people have all the fun. The implication is that you shouldn't be nice if you want to find a relationship. In truth, the quality of being nice is among the most highly valued in potential partners.

KIM IS A social worker in Chicago. "I was set up on a blind date. I was a little hesitant at first because I had never been on a blind date before, and I wasn't quite sure what to expect," Kim says.

"We spoke on the telephone a few times and had good conversations. He was very much into music. I told him I like all kinds of music, but I was getting more and more into jazz. He invited me on a jazz cruise, and I accepted. He seemed kind of nice, so I bought a bottle of cheap champagne and two plastic cups for the date.

"When I got into his car, he had a bag. It was Moët and real champagne glasses. I laughed to myself, but I didn't tell him why I was laughing. It was a nice surprise. I never did pull out my $7.99 bottle.

"When we got to the pier, we opened the champagne and had a toast to new friendships and new beginnings. The boat ride was romantic. He was not trying to kiss me or anything like that. It was just a nice wholesome date with a nice guy."

Looking back after three years of marriage, Kim remembers her trepidation about the blind date and says, "Don't let anybody tell you there aren't any nice guys out there."

Among those seeking a relationship, the degree to which a potential partner was nice and kind was a significant factor for more than 75 percent of respondents. (Herold and Milhausen 1999)

Your Goals Must Engage All of You

To pursue something difficult, you will need commitment, focus, confidence. You will need the promise of gaining a significant outcome and a sense of fulfillment. If your goals do not move you, if they do not inspire and incite you to action, then you have not found the right goals.

LACEY BENTON HAS worked for, and run, a long list of small businesses in the Baltimore area. Unfortunately, after a while she would realize her heart wasn't in it.

While Lacey had enjoyed working with youth groups, she never saw the possibility of making a career out of her efforts. That was until a community center called the Village Learning Place invited her to oversee their plans to rent out part of their building to create a small café.

Then Lacey took the conversation in a whole new direction: "You have teenagers here looking for something worthwhile to do, and you have a space you'd like to rent to generate some income. Forget about renting it. Let's create a café ourselves," Lacey told the group's board. She proposed letting the teens be involved in every aspect of the operation. She would use her years of small-business experience to make sure it ran smoothly.

The idea of teaching business skills to teens was so intriguing that the center was able to attract grant money to help open the Youth Entrepreneur Café.

Lacey loves working with young people as they gain a sense of accomplishment from the café. As for Lacey, when the mind and heart are focused on the same thing, "I can do anything. Watch me," she says.

When end-of-career managers discussed their relative success and moments of peak performance during their careers, more than half spoke in terms of the significance of personal fulfillment. (Thornton, Privette, and Bundrick 1999)

See the Horizon, and Watch Your Step

Relationships are built on long-term values and short-term actions. A long-term perspective will give your relationship value to you in the moment, which is where you need to demonstrate, on a day-to-day, moment-to-moment basis, your dedication to a healthy relationship. As is the case with anything you really want in life, you need to see the long-term hope and the short-term need.

FAMED PHOTOGRAPHER ALFRED Stieglitz was unhappy when his wife, painter Georgia O'Keeffe, kept talking about spending summers in the Southwest. He much preferred his family's retreat at Lake George in upstate New York. Finally, she decided to go on her own.

Georgia O'Keeffe said her first summer in the Southwest was "bliss" and that she'd "never felt better in my life." But Alfred did not see it that way. He called it "maybe the most trying" experience of his life. But he did take a lot more photographs of her when she got back from that first trip. More than he had in years.

The notion of a marriage sabbatical—time away from one's partner to refresh oneself—has advocates among psychologists. "It's not for everyone," psychologist Penelope Sanders says. "If you don't have a burning desire to write or hike the Appalachian trail, that's just fine. I'm not advocating that every married person take off but that we broaden our ideas of what's possible in marriage.

"Whenever you do something alone and something hard, and you do it well, you can't help but feel really good about yourself and about life," Penelope says. "And those feelings spill over to your relationship."

People in satisfying relationships were five times more likely to have a long-term perspective on their lives, actively thinking about the long-term future, than a short-term perspective. (Arriaga and Agnew 2001)

Follow Through for You

People who do what they say they are going to do tend to be healthier than less reliable people. The attitude that allows us to commit and to exhibit a sense of control contributes to our ability not only to follow health advice but to believe in our own health. Develop a long-standing habit of reliability, and benefits for your health and your life will follow.

PSYCHOLOGY PROFESSOR ALAN Christensen of the University of Iowa has found that our attitudes and approaches to life matter to our health. "You will be better off if you're conscientious," he says.

"Conscientiousness refers to diligence, a strong sense of personal control, and a willingness to take on personal challenges," he adds. "In short, it is a commitment to follow the course you set yourself on without reluctance.

"It may be as important to think about patients' psychological traits, emotions and behaviors, and how they see and approach the world and themselves as it is to consider the physical status of the patient," Professor Christensen says. "We all know people who tend toward anxiety or inaction. Typically we just think, 'Oh, that's just how they are.' But we should be paying attention, because these traits could be shortening their lives."

Although we don't usually think of such lifelong, enduring traits as being easy to change, Professor Christensen says there is reason to believe individuals can alter their degree of conscientiousness. Moreover, doctors should be able to use information about how their patients' personalities may be putting them at risk to judge how closely they need to be monitored and how aggressively to treat them.

In a study of those suffering a chronic illness, researchers found that those who tended to be highly conscientious, goal directed, and dependable were 36 percent less likely to die prematurely. (University of Iowa 2002b)

Only You Can Say If
This Is a World You Can Succeed In

Those who lack confidence pay attention to those who have failed and to the obstacles that exist to thwart their own efforts. The confident see a reality in which success is possible because they pay special attention to those who have succeeded and have carefully studied the path to success.

PRIME MINISTER WINSTON Churchill, who led Great Britain through World War II, is thought of by many experts as being perhaps the best example of a person who led a complete life and functioned to the best of all his abilities. Churchill not only led a government through the most overwhelming circumstance but spent his life engaged in such pursuits as studying, painting, writing, and raising a family.

However, one year after the treaties were signed that ended all hostilities in the war, Winston Churchill was voted out of office. He left office shocked and humbled and feeling himself a failure.

By no reasonable standard would Winston Churchill have to accomplish so much to be considered a success. But at the same time, by only one standard could Winston Churchill consider himself a success. If Churchill did not see himself as having succeeded, then no accomplishment would suffice.

Research on middle-class men from similar backgrounds finds that they have a greatly divergent view of how difficult it is to succeed economically. Despite the fact that their lives had similar economic and social challenges, some viewed the world as tilted against them, while others saw it as offering great opportunities. The more optimistically they viewed their surroundings, the greater their satisfaction with their jobs and their confidence in future success. (Franklin and Mizell 1995)

There's No Deadline for Your Dreams

Live your life toward your dreams. No one will ask you what date it is when you get there.

HE HAS SPENT twenty years in the military. He's married and has six children. He drives a minivan. And he's playing college football for the University of South Carolina.

Tim Frisby went straight into the military after high school. He loved sports as a child and would have loved to go to college, but he felt the military was his best career opportunity. Throughout his two decades of military service, he followed college football and his favorite team, South Carolina.

As an army ranger, fitness was a constant part of his life, but he often thought of the day his military career would be over. "I dreamed of playing college football. It was in the back of my head every day," Tim says.

His teammates have nicknamed him "Pops." But Tim says that although he's "older than some of my teammates' parents," he spends not a moment wishing he was younger.

Tim's not out to prove a point, either. "I don't want to be a novelty," he says. "I don't want to be sitting on the sidelines with the only thing people saying is 'That guy is thirty-nine, but he's not really contributing.' I want to contribute."

South Carolina coaches rave about his attitude, his commitment, his work ethic, and his leadership abilities. "He sets an example for his teammates every day," one assistant coach says.

His military colleagues think he sets a shining example for them, too. "You're never too old to reach your goals," says one of his officers. "Tim's definitely a morale builder for these soldiers."

People who feel they have reached their life dream are more likely to feel satisfied with their life, but the age at which they reached their dream is unrelated to their satisfaction. (Krueger 1998)

Sources

Acitelli, L, D. Kenny, and D. Weiner. 2001. "The Importance of Similarity and Understanding of Partners' Marital Ideals to Relationship Satisfaction." *Personal Relationships* 8:167–85.

Alderman, M. K. 1999. *Motivation for Achievement: Possibilities for Teaching and Learning.* Mahwah, NJ: Lawrence Erlbaum Associates.

Allen, S., and P. Webster. 2001. "When Wives Get Sick: Gender Role Attitude, Marital Happiness, and Husbands' Contribution to Household Labor." *Gender and Society* 15:898–916.

American Academy of Orthopaedic Surgeons. 2002. "When Traveling, Leave the Extra Baggage at Home."

American College of Allergy, Asthma and Immunology. 2002. "Allergies Interfere with Life."

Appleton, C., and E. Bohm. 2001. "Partners in Passage: The Experience of Marriage in Mid-Life." *Journal of Phenomenological Psychology* 32:41–70.

Arnett, J. 2000. "High Hopes in a Grim World." *Youth and Society* 31:267–86.

Arnold, K. 1995. *Lives of Promise: A Fourteen-Year Study of Achievement and Life Choices.* San Francisco: Jossey-Bass.

Arriaga, X., and C. Agnew. 2001. "Being Committed: Affective, Cognitive, and Conative Components of Relationship Commitment." *Personality and Social Psychology Bulletin* 27:1190–1203.

Arrison, E. 1998. "Academic Self-Confidence as a Predictor of First-Year College Student Quality of Effort and Achievement." Ph.D. dissertation, Temple University.

Atkinson, S. 1999. "Reflections: Personal Development for Managers." *Journal of Managerial Psychology* 14:502–11.

Auerbach, S., A. Penberthy, and D. Kiesler. 2004. "Opportunity for Control, Interpersonal Impacts, and Adjustment to a Long-Term Invasive Health Care Procedure." *Journal of Behavioral Medicine* 27 (1): 11–29.

Austin, L. 2000. *What's Holding You Back?* New York: Basic Books.

Azarow, J. 2003. "Generativity and Well-Being: An Investigation of the Eriksonian Hypothesis." Ph.D. dissertation, Northwestern University.

Bachand, L., and S. Caron. 2001. "Ties That Bind: A Qualitative Study of Happy Long-Term Marriages." *Contemporary Family Therapy* 21:105–21.

Baker, B. 2000. "Responses to Dependence: A Social Exchange Model of Employment Practices in Entrepreneurial Firms." Ph.D. dissertation, University of North Carolina.

Bargdill, R. 1998. "Being Bored with One's Life: An Empirical Phenomenological Study." Ph.D. dissertation, Duquesne University.

———. 2000. "The Study of Life Boredom." *Journal of Phenomenological Psychology* 31 (2): 188–219.

Barile, C. 2001. "The Never-Married, Caucasian, American Woman in Mid-Life as a Departure from the Stereotypes of the Old Maid Spinster." Ph.D. dissertation, Pacifica Graduate Institute.

Barofsky, I., and A. Rowan. 1998. "Models for Measuring Quality of Life: Implications for Human-Animal Interaction Research." In *Companion Animals in Human Health.* Thousand Oaks, CA: Sage.

Barto, V. 1998. "The Relationship Between Personality Traits of Selected New Jersey Public High School Educators and Successful Academic Achievement of At-Risk Students." Ph.D. dissertation, Seton Hall University.

Bashaw, R. E., and E. S. Grant. 1994. "Exploring the Distinctive Nature of Work Commitments." *Journal of Personal Selling and Sales Management* 14:41–56.

Berry, J., and E. Worthington. 2001. "Forgivingness, Relationship Quality, Stress While Imagining Relationship Events, and Physical and Mental Health." *Journal of Counseling Psychology* 48:447–55.

Black, H. 1999. "A Sense of the Sacred: Altering or Enhancing the Self-Portrait in Older Age?" *Narrative Inquiry* 9:327–45.

Boehne, D., and P. Pease. 2000. "Deciding Whether to Complete or Terminate an Unfinished Project." *Organizational Behavior and Human Decision Processes* 81:178–94.

Bonds-Raacke, J., E. Bearden, N. Carriere, E. Anderson, and S. Nicks. 2001. "Engaging Distortions: Are We Idealizing Marriage?" *Journal of Psychology* 135:179–84.

Boyer, G. 1999. "Turning Points in the Development of Male Servant Leaders." Ph.D. dissertation, Fielding Institute.

Boyer-Pennington, M., J. Pennington, and C. Spink. 2001. "Students' Expectations and Optimism Toward Marriage as a Function of Parental Divorce." *Journal of Divorce and Remarriage* 34:71–87.

Brady, E. M., and H. Sky. 2003. "Journal Writing Among Older Adults." *Educational Gerontology* 29:151–63.

Brebner, J., 1995. "Testing for Stress and Happiness: The Role of Personality Factors." In *Stress and Emotion: Anxiety, Anger, and Curiosity.* Washington, DC: Taylor and Francis.

Brigham Young University. 2002. "Spouses Often Mirror Each Others' Health."

Brown, J., and K. Dutton. 1995. "The Thrill of Victory, the Complexity of Defeat: Self-Esteem and People's Emotional Reaction to Success and Failure." *Journal of Personality and Social Psychology* 68:712.

Brown, S. 1999. "Holding Up a Mirror: Identity Revision and Its Relationship to Women's Voluntary Career Change." Ph.D. dissertation, Fielding Institute.

Brown University. 2002. "Personality as Heart Disease Risk Factor."

Burack, O., P. Jefferson, and L. Libow. 2002. "Individualized Music: A Route to

Improving the Quality of Life for Long-Term Care Residents." *Activities, Adaptation and Aging* 27 (1): 63–76.

Bush, H., R. Williams, M. Lean, and A. Anderson. 2001. "Body Image and Weight Consciousness Among South Asian, Italian, and General Population Women in Britain." *Appetite* 37:207–15.

Butler, R. 1999. "Information Seeking and Achievement Motivation in Middle Childhood and Adolescence: The Role of Conceptions of Ability." *Developmental Psychology* 35:146–63.

Bybee, J., S. Luthar, and E. Zigler. 1997. "The Fantasy, Ideal, and Ought Selves." *Social Cognition* 15:37–53.

Cambridge University. 2002. "Low Vitamin C Intake Linked with Stroke Risk."

Cameron, P. 1972. "Stereotypes About Generational Fun and Happiness vs. Self-Appraised Fun and Happiness." *Gerontologist* 12 (2): 120–23.

Carpenter, S. 2000. "Effects of Cultural Tightness and Collectivism on Self-Concept and Causal Attributions." *Social Science* 34:38–56.

Carsten, K. 2001. "Enhancing Satisfaction Through Downward Comparison: The Role of Relational Discontent and Individual Differences in Social Comparison Orientation." *Journal of Experimental Social Psychology* 37:452–67.

Case Western Reserve University. 2002. "More Exercise, Less Smoking May Extend, Enhance Life Even at Advanced Age."

Case Western Reserve University School of Medicine. 2002. "Television and the Brain."

Caughlin, J., and T. Golish. 2002. "An Analysis of the Association Between Topic Avoidance and Dissatisfaction: Comparing Perceptual and Interpersonal Explanations." *Communication Monographs* 69 (4): 275–95.

Caughlin, J., and T. Huston. 2002. "A Contextual Analysis of the Association Between Demand/Withdraw and Marital Satisfaction." *Personal Relationships* 9:95–119.

Centers for Disease Control and Prevention. 2000. "Skip the Elevator."

Chamberlain, J., and D. Haaga. 2001. "Unconditional Self-Acceptance and Psychological Health." *Journal of Rational-Emotive and Cognitive Behavior Therapy* 19 (3): 163–76.

Chambers, J., and P. Windschitl. 2004. "Biases in Social Comparative Judgments: The Role of Nonmotivated Factors in Above-Average and Comparative-Optimism Effects." *Psychological Bulletin* 130:813–38.

Chen, Y., and B. King. 2002. "Intra- and Intergenerational Communication Satisfaction as a Function of an Individual's Age and Age Stereotypes." *International Journal of Behavioral Development* 26 (6): 562–70.

Childs, B. G. 1998. "Academically Gifted Girls." Ph.D. dissertation, Case Western Reserve University.

Chou, K, and I. Chi. 2001. "Stressful Life Events and Depressive Symptoms: Social Support and Sense of Control as Mediators or Moderators?" *International Journal of Aging and Human Development* 52:155–71.

Christiansen, C. 2000. "Identity, Personal Projects and Happiness: Self-Construction in Everyday Action." *Journal of Occupational Science* 7 (3): 98–107.

Cincinnati Children's Hospital. 2002. "Study Warns of Eating Meals in Front of TV."

Clarke, S. 1998. "Taking Care: Women High School Teachers at Midlife and Midcareer." Ph.D. dissertation, University of Massachusetts.

Cohan, C., and S. Cole. 2002. "Life Course Transitions and Natural Disaster: Marriage, Birth, and Divorce Following Hurricane Hugo." *Journal of Family Psychology* 16:14–25.

Colorado State University. 2002. "Choosing the Right Drink for Fluid Replacement."

Columbia University. 2003a. "Effects on Cognitive Ability of Sedentary Lifestyle."

———. 2003b. "Religiosity Effect on Mental Health."

Columbus Children's Hospital. 2002. "Smoking Outside Still Causes Second-Hand Smoke Exposure to Children."

Conway, C. 2000. "Using the Crucial Cs to Explore Gender Roles with Couples." *Journal of Individual Psychology* 56:495–501.

Cooper, B., P. Clasen, D. Silva-Jalonen, and M. Butler. 1999. "Creative Performance on an In-Basket Exercise." *Journal of Managerial Psychology* 14:39–56.

Coover, G., and S. Murphy. 2000. "The Communicated Self: Exploring the Interaction Between Self and Social Context." *Human Communication Research* 26:125–47.

Cornell University. 2001. "Mothers Who Lose Weight After the Birth of Their First Child Have a 'Can Do' Attitude."

Cornell University. 2002a. "Lycopene Effects."

———. 2002b. "Noise Impairments."

Coulthard, P. 1998. "The Quality-Achieving Behavior of Work Group Managers." Ph.D. dissertation, Portland State University.

Cox, D. 2001. "'Smile, Honey, Our Church Is Watching': Identity and Role Conflict in the Pastoral Marriage." Ph.D. dissertation, University of South Florida.

Crosnoe, R., and G. Elder. 2002. "Successful Adaptation in the Later Years: A Life Course Approach to Aging." *Social Psychology Quarterly* 65:309–28.

Dana-Farber Cancer Institute. 2002. "Large Doses of Vitamins and Minerals May Put Prostate Cancer Patients at Risk."

Dana-Farber Center for Community Based Research. 2002. "Worksite Program to Stop Smoking Among Blue-Collar Workers Yields Notable Success."

Dartmouth Medical School. 2003. "More Health Care Doesn't Equal Better Health Care."

Decker, W., and D. Rotondo. 1999. "Use of Humor at Work: Predictors and Implications." *Psychological Reports* 84:961–68.

De Koning, E., and R. Weiss. 2002. "The Relational Humor Inventory: Functions of Humor in Close Relationships." *American Journal of Family Therapy* 30:1–18.

DeShon, R., and J. Gillespie. 2005. "A Motivated Action Theory Account of Goal Orientation." Journal of Applied Psychology 90:1096–1127.

Dickinson, M. J. 1999. "Do Gooders or Do Betters?" *Educational Research* 41:221–27.

Diener, E., and F. Fujita. 1995. "Resources, Personal Strivings, and Subjective Well-Being." *Journal of Personality and Social Psychology* 68:926.

Diener, E., and M. Suh. 1998. "Subjective Well-Being and Age: An International Analysis." *Annual Review of Gerontology and Geriatrics* 17:304–24

Dorfman, D. 2001. "The Impact of Mother's Work on the Life Choices and Sense of Self of the Young Adult Daughter During Motherhood: A Self-Psychological Perspective." Ph.D. dissertation, New York University.

Drigotas, S., C. Rusbult, and J. Verette. 1999. "Level of Commitment, Mutuality of Commitment, and Couple Well-Being." *Personal Relationships* 6:389–409.

Dube, L., M. Jodoin, and S. Kairouz. 1998. "On the Cognitive Basis of Subjective Well-Being Analysis: What Do Individuals Have to Say About It?" *Canadian Journal of Behavioural Science* 30 (1): 1–13.

Dufore, S. 2000. "Marital Similarity, Marital Interaction, and Couples' Shared View of Their Marriage." Ph.D. dissertation, Syracuse University.

Duke University. 2002. "Effects of Stress Management on Patient Recovery."

Duke University. 2003. "Distance to Treatment Center and Mastectomy vs. Lumpectomy."

Easterlin, R. 2001. "Life Cycle Welfare: Evidence and Conjecture." *Journal of Socio-Economics* 30 (1): 31–61.

Ebesu Hubbard, A. 2001. "Conflict Between Relationally Uncertain Romantic Partners: The Influence of Relational Responsiveness and Empathy." *Communication Monographs* 68:400–414.

Efklides, A., M. Kalaitzidou, and G. Chankin. 2003. "Subjective Quality of Life in Old Age in Greece: The Effect of Demographic Factors, Emotional State and Adaptation to Aging." *European Psychologist* 8 (3): 178–91.

Eisenberger, R., L. Rhoades, and J. Cameron. 1999. "Does Pay for Performance Increase or Decrease Perceived Self-Determination and Intrinsic Motivation?" *Journal of Personality and Social Psychology* 77:1026–40.

Eldridge, K. 2001. "Demand-Withdraw Communication During Marital Conflict: Relationship Satisfaction and Gender Role Considerations." Ph.D. dissertation, University of California, Los Angeles.

Elliott, M. 1999. "Time, Work, and Meaning." Ph.D. dissertation, Pacifica Graduate Institute.

Emory University. 2002a. "Majority of U.S. Adults Have Some Health Problems."

———. 2002b. "Pesticide Exposure Linked to Parkinson's."

Erdwins, C., L. Buffardi, W. Casper, and A. O'Brien. 2001. "The Relationship of Women's Role Strain to Social Support, Role Satisfaction, and Self-Efficacy." *Family Relations* 50:230–38.

Fahrenkamp, E. 2001. "Age, Gender, and Perceived Social Support of Married and Never-Married Persons as Predictors of Self-Esteem." Ph.D. dissertation, Texas A&M University.

Fallon, J., J. Avis, J. Kudisch, T. Gornet, and A. Frost. 2000. "Conscientiousness as a Predictor of Productive and Counterproductive Behaviors." *Journal of Business and Psychology* 15:339–49.

Feather, N. T. 1999. "Judgments of Deservingness: Studies in the Psychology of Justice and Achievement." *Personality and Social Psychology Review* 3:86–107.

Felmlee, D. 2001. "From Appealing to Appalling: Disenchantment with a Romantic Partner." *Sociological Perspectives* 44:263–80.

Fisher, S., W. D. K. Macrosson, and J. Wong. 1998. "Cognitive Style and Team Role Preference." *Journal of Managerial Psychology* 13:544–57.

Fisk, A. 2002. "Can Marital Interaction Predict Women's Relapse After Dieting?" Ph.D. dissertation, Alliant International University.

Fitness, J. 2001. "Emotional Intelligence and Intimate Relationships." In *Emotional Intelligence in Everyday Life: A Scientific Inquiry*, ed. J. Ciarrochi and J. Forgas. New York: Psychology Press.

Flett, G., P. Hewitt, B. Shapiro, and J. Rayman. 2002. "Perfectionism, Beliefs, and Adjustment in Dating Relationships." *Current Psychology* 20:289–311.

Food and Drug Administration. 2002. "Physicians Honor Patient Requests for Advertised Drugs."

Fowers, B. 2001. "The Limits of Technical Concept of a Good Marriage: Exploring the Role of Virtue in Communication Skills." *Journal of Marital and Family Therapy* 27:327–40.

Fowers, B., E. Lyons, K. Montel, and N. Shaked. 2001. "Positive Illusions About Marriage Among Married and Single Individuals." *Journal of Family Psychology* 15:95–109.

Francis, L., S. Jones, and C. Wilcox. 2000. "Religiosity and Happiness: During Adolescence, Young Adulthood, and Later Life." *Journal of Psychology and Christianity* 19 (3): 245–57.

Franklin, C. W., and C. A. Mizell. 1995. "Some Factors Influencing Success Among African American Men." *Journal of Men's Studies* 3:191–204.

Freed, D. 2004. "Material Benefits, Advancement, or Fulfillment: A Study into the Causes and Predictors of Job Satisfaction Based on How People View Their Work." Ph.D. dissertation, Nova Southeastern University.

Freeman, L. D. Templer, and C. Hill. 1999. "The Relationship Between Adult Happiness and Self-Appraised Childhood Happiness and Events." *Journal of Genetic Psychology* 160 (1): 46–54.

Frey, B., and A. Stutzer. 2000. "Happiness Prospers in Democracy." *Journal of Happiness Studies* 1 (3): 79–102.

Frijters, P. 2000. "Do Individuals Try to Maximize General Satisfaction?" *Journal of Economic Psychology* 21 (3): 281–304.

Frome, P. 1999. "The Influence of Girls' Gender-Linked Beliefs on Their Educational and Occupational Aspirations." Ph.D. dissertation, University of Michigan.

Gerdtham, U., and M. Johannesson. 2001. "The Relationship Between Happiness, Health, and Social Economic Factors." *Journal of Socio-Economics* 30 (6): 553–57.

Gilbert, L., and S. Walker. 2001. "Contemporary Marriage." In *The New Handbook of Psychotherapy and Counseling with Men*, ed. G. Brooks and G. Glenn. San Francisco: Jossey-Bass.

Glaman, J. 1999. "Competitiveness and the Similarity-Attraction Effect Among Co-Workers." Ph.D. dissertation, University of Houston.

Glasman, L. 2002. "Mother 'There for' Me: Female-Identity Development in the Context of the Mother-Daughter Relationship. A Qualitative Study." Ph.D. dissertation, New York University.

Goldenberg, S., and T. Kline. 1999. "An Exploratory Study of Predicting Perceived Success and Survival of Small Businesses." *Psychological Reports* 85:365–77.

Goldscheider, F. 2001. "Men's Changing Family Relationships." In *Couples in Conflict*, ed. A. Booth, A. Crouter, and M. Clements. Mahwah, NJ: Lawrence Erlbaum Associates.

Goltz, S. 1999. "Can't Stop on a Dime: The Roles of Matching and Momentum in Persistence of Commitment." *Journal of Organizational Behavior Management* 19:37–63.

Gordon, Darlene. 1998. "The Relationship Among Academic Self-Concept, Academic Achievement, and Persistence with Self-Attribution." Ph.D. dissertation, Purdue University.

Gotlib, I., E. Krasnoperova, D. N. Yue, and J. Joormann. 2004. "Attentional Biases for Negative Interpersonal Stimuli in Clinical Depression." *Journal of Abnormal Psychology* 113 (1): 121–35.

Goulet, L., and P. Singh. 2002. "Career Commitment: A Reexamination and an Extension." *Journal of Vocational Behavior* 61:73–91.

Green, M., J. Hilken, H. Friedman, K. Grossman, J. Gasiewski, R. Adler, and J. Sabini. 2005. "Communication via Instant Messenger: Short- and Long-Term Effects." *Journal of Applied Social Psychology* 35:487–507.

Greene, A. 1999. "Honesty in Organizations: Perceptions of the Corporate Environment and Their Impact on Individual Behavior." Ph.D. dissertation, Brandeis University.

Greno-Malsch, K. L. 1998. "Children's Use of Interpersonal Negotiation Strategies as a Function of Their Level of Self-Worth." Ph.D. dissertation, University of Wisconsin–Milwaukee.

Gribble, J. R. 2000. "The Psychosocial Crisis of Industry Versus Inferiority and Self-Estimates of Vocational Competence in High School Students." Ph.D. dissertation, Kent State University.

Guerra, A., and J. Braungart-Rieker. 1999. "Predicting Career Indecision in College Students." *Career Development Quarterly* 47:255–66.

Hackensack University Medical Center. 1999. "Regular Soap Safer Than Antibacterial Soap."

Hagan, C. 1999. "The Relationship Between Employee Job Satisfaction and Key Customer Outcomes." Ph.D. dissertation, Florida Atlantic University.

Hairston, R. 2001. "Predicting Marital Satisfaction Among African American Couples." Ph.D. dissertation, Seattle Pacific University.

Hamarat, E., D. Thompson, K. Zabrucky, and D. Steele. 2001. "Perceived Stress and Coping Resource Availability as Predictors of Life Satisfaction in Young, Middle-Aged, and Older Adults." *Experimental Aging Research* 27 (2): 181–96.

Harris, K. 2001. "The Psychophysiology of Marital Interaction: Differential Effects of Support and Conflict." Ph.D. dissertation, University of Oregon.

Harrison, Y., and J. Horne. 1999. "One Night of Sleep Loss Impairs Innovative Thinking and Flexible Decision Making." *Organizational Behavior and Human Decision Processes* 78:128–45.

Hart, P. 1999. "Predicting Employee Life Satisfaction: A Coherent Model of Personality, Work, and Nonwork Experiences, and Domain Satisfactions." *Journal of Applied Psychology* 84 (4): 564–84.

Harvard University. 2003. "Breathing and Blood Flow."

Haugen, R., and T. Lund. 1999. "The Concept of General Expectancy in Various Personality Dispositions." *Scandinavian Journal of Psychology* 40:109–14.

Henderson, E. 1999. "Extensive Engagement: Chief Executive Officers' Formative Life Experiences Related to Their Participative Style of Leadership." Ph.D. dissertation, University of Alberta.

Herold, E., and R. Milhausen. 1999. "Dating Preferences of University Women: An Analysis of the Nice Guy Stereotype." *Journal of Sex and Marital Therapy* 25:333–43.

Hills, P., and M. Argyle. 2001. "Emotional Stability as a Major Dimension of Happiness." *Personality and Individual Differences* 31 (8): 1357–64.

Hoeveler, F. 1999. "Attachment Style and Mother-Daughter Conflict at the Beginning of Adolescence." Ph.D. dissertation, Antioch University.

Housker, J. 2001. "Houston's Model of Guided Imagery Combined with Music: Strengthening Couples' Relationships." Ph.D. dissertation, University of South Dakota.

Howatt, W. A. 1999. "Journaling to Self-Evaluation: A Tool for Adult Learners." *International Journal of Reality Therapy* 18:32–34.

Huston, T. 2000. "The Social Ecology of Marriage and Other Intimate Unions." *Journal of Marriage and the Family* 62:298–319.

Huston, T., J. Caughlin, R. Houts, S. Smith, and L. George. 2001. "The Connubial Crucible: Newlywed Years as Predictors of Marital Delight, Distress, and Divorce." *Journal of Personality and Social Psychology* 80:237–52.

Ichniowski, C., D. Levine, C. Olsen, and G. Strauss. 2000. *The American Workplace: Skills, Compensation, and Employee Involvement.* New York: Cambridge University Press.

Ikeuchi, H., and T. Fujihara. 2000. "The Effects of Loss of Material Possessions and Social Support Network on the Quality of Life." *Japanese Journal of Social Psychology* 16 (2): 92–102.

Ingram, M. P. B. 1998. "A Study of Transformative Aspects of Career Change Experiences and Implications for Current Models of Career Development." Ph.D. dissertation, Texas A&M University.

Isaacowitz, D., G. Vaillant, and M. Seligman. 2003. "Strengths and Satisfaction Across the Adult Lifespan." *International Journal of Aging and Human Development* 57 (2): 181–201.

Jackson, S., L. Mayocchi, and J. Dover. 1998. "Life After Winning Gold." *Sport Psychologist* 12:137–55.

Janoff-Bulman, R., and H. Leggatt. 2002. "Culture and Social Obligation: When 'Shoulds' Are Perceived as 'Wants.'" *Journal of Research in Personality* 36:260–70.

Jeffres, L., and J. Dobos. 1995. "Separating People's Satisfaction with Life and Public Perceptions of the Quality of Life in the Environment." *Social Indicators Research* 34:181.

Johns Hopkins University. 1997. "The Pace of Eating."

Johnson, M., T. Beebe, J. Mortimer, and M. Snyder. 1998. "Volunteerism in Adolescence: A Process Perspective." *Journal of Research on Adolescence* 8:309–32.

Johnson, M., B. Karney, R. Rogge, and T. Bradbury. 2001. "The Role of Marital Behavior in the Longitudinal Association Between Attributions and Marital Quality." In *Attribution, Communication Behavior, and Close Relationships,* ed. V. Manusov and J. Harvey. New York: Cambridge University Press.

Jokisaari, M. 2003. "Regret Appraisals, Age, and Subjective Well-Being." *Journal of Research in Personality* 37 (6): 487–503.

Jones, D. 2000. "Appreciative Inquiry." Ph.D. dissertation, Benedictine University.

Jones, E., and S. Berglas. 1999. "Control of the Attributions About the Self Through Self-Handicapping Strategies." In *The Self in Social Psychology,* ed. R. Baumeister. Philadelphia: Taylor and Francis.

Juang, L., and R. Silbereisen. 2001. "Family Transitions for Young Adult Women." *American Behavioral Scientist* 44:1899–1917.

Judge, T., C. Thoresen, V. Pucik, and T. Welbourne. 1999. "Managerial Coping with Organizational Change." *Journal of Applied Psychology* 84:107–22.

Karney, B., and N. Frye. 2002. "But We've Been Getting Better Lately": Comparing Prospective and Retrospective Views of Relationship Development." *Journal of Personality and Social Psychology* 82:222–38.

Kelly, A., and J. Carter. 2001. "Dealing with Secrets." In *Coping with Stress: Effective People and Processes,* ed. C. Snyder. New York: Oxford University Press.

King, L., and C. Napa. 1998. "What Makes a Life Good?" *Journal of Personality and Social Psychology* 75:156–65.

Kinnier, R., N. Tribbensee, C. Rose, and S. Vaughan. 2001. "In the Final Analysis: More Wisdom from People Who Have Faced Death." *Journal of Counseling and Development* 79 (2): 171–77.

Klute, M., A. Crouter, A. Sayer, and S. McHale. 2002. "Occupational Self-Direction, Values, and Egalitarian Relationships: A Study of Dual-Earner Couples." *Journal of Marriage and the Family* 64:139–51.

Knouse, S., J. Tanner, and E. Harris. 1999. "The Relation of College Internships, College Performance, and Subsequent Job Opportunity." *Journal of Employment Counseling* 36:35–43.

Knox, D., and M. Zusman. 2001. "Marrying a Man with 'Baggage': Implications for Second Wives." *Journal of Divorce and Remarriage* 35:67–79.

Koehne, K. 2000. "The Relationship Between Relational Commitment, Spousal Intimacy, and Religiosity and Marital Satisfaction." Ph.D. dissertation, University of Tennessee.

Korn, A. 2002. "Motherhood: An Exploration of Changes in the Mother-Daughter Relationship." Ph.D. dissertation, Adelphi University.

Kroth, J., A. Daline, D. Longstreet, M. Nelson, and L. O'Neal. 2002. "Sleep, Dreams, and Job Satisfaction." *Psychological Reports* 90 (3): 876–78.

Krueger, R. 1998. "The Status of Perceived Dream Fulfillment in Midlife Males." Ph.D. dissertation, California School of Professional Psychology.

Kulik, L. 2001. "The Impact of Men's and Women's Retirement on Marital Relations: A Comparative Analysis." *Journal of Women and Aging* 13:21–37.

Larsen, J., A. P. McGraw, and J. Cacioppo. 2001. "Can People Feel Happy and Sad at the Same Time?" *Journal of Personality and Social Psychology* 81 (4): 684–96.

Lawrence, T. 2001. "Secure Base Behaviors and Mental Representations of Attachment in Early Marriage." Ph.D. dissertation, State University of New York at Stony Brook.

Leader, J. 2001. "Family Defense Styles and Their Relationship to Family Functioning." Ph.D. dissertation, Boston University.

LeSure-Lester, G. 2001. "Dating Competence, Social Assertion and Social Anxiety Among College Students." *College Student Journal* 35:317–20.

Levine, S. 2000. "Gender Differences in Loneliness and Marital Quality in Young Married Couples." Ph.D. dissertation, California School of Professional Psychology.

Lindeman, M., and M. Verkasalo. 1996. "Meaning in Life." *Journal of Social Psychology* 136:657.

Lockhart, A. 2000. "Perceived Influence of a Disney Fairy Tale on Beliefs About Romantic Love and Marriage." Ph.D. dissertation, California School of Professional Psychology.

Lockwood, P., and Z. Kunda. 2000. "Outstanding Role Models: Do They Inspire or Demoralize Us?" In *Psychological Perspectives on Self and Identity,* ed. A. Tesser. Washington, DC: American Psychological Association.

Lomas, P. 2004. *Wonder and the Loss of Wonder.* Philadelphia: Whurr Publishers.

Lounsbury, J., J. Loveland, E. Sundstrom, and L. Gibson. 2003. "An Investigation of Personality Traits in Relation to Career Satisfaction." *Journal of Career Assessment* 11 (3): 287–307.

Loveless, A. 2000. "Paired Conceptions of Morality and Happiness as Factors in Marital Happiness." Ph.D. dissertation, Brigham Young University.

Lucas, J., and R. Heady. 2002. "Flextime Commuters and Their Driver Stress, Feelings of Time Urgency, and Commute Satisfaction." *Journal of Business and Psychology* 16 (4): 565–72.

Ludlow, L., and R. Alvarez-Salvat. 2001. "Spillover in the Academy: Marriage Stability and Faculty Evaluations." *Journal of Personal Evaluation in Education* 15:111–19.

Ludwig, K. 2000. "Responses to Dissatisfaction: An Integrative Analysis of Change Attempts and Relationship Quality." Ph.D. dissertation, Auburn University.

Lyubomirsky, S., L. King, and E. Diener. 2005. "The Benefits of Frequent Positive Affect: Does Happiness Lead to Success?" *Psychological Bulletin* 131:803–55.

Maasen, G., and J. Landsheer. 2000. "Peer-Perceived Social Competence and Academic Achievement of Low-Level Educated Young Adolescents." *Social Behavior and Personality* 28:29–40.

Maltby, J., L. Day, and L. Barber. 2005. "Forgiveness and Happiness, the Differing Contexts of Forgiveness Using the Distinction Between Hedonic and Eudaimonic Happiness." *Journal of Happiness Studies* 6:1–13.

Marks, S., T. Huston, E. Johnson, and S. MacDermid. 2001. "Role Balance Among White Married Couples." *Journal of Marriage and the Family* 63:1083–98.

Mayo, M. W., and N. Christenfeld. 1999. "Gender, Race, and Performance Expectations of College Students." *Journal of Multicultural Counseling and Development* 27:93–104.

Mayo Clinic. 2002a. "An Aspirin a Day to Keep Cancer Away?"

———. 2002b. "Only Five to 10 Percent of Cancers Are Inherited."

———. 2002c. "Optimism and Life Expectancy."

———. 2002d. "Toothbrush and Floss Compare Well to Electric Versions."

———. 2003. "Household Mold Scares: Small Amounts Not a Big Health Concern."

McAuley, E., B. Blissmer, D. Marquez, and G. Jerome. 2000. "Social Relations, Physical Activity and Well-Being in Older Adults." *Preventive Medicine* 31 (5): 608–17.

McCarter, J. 2000. "Adult Daughters' Reflections on Mother: Weaving a Separate Self." Ph.D. dissertation, University of Nebraska.

McCaw, W. 1999. "The Perception of Followers." Ph.D. dissertation, University of Montana.

McGregor, I. D. 1999. "An Identity Consolidation View of Social Phenomena: Theory and Research." Ph.D. dissertation, University of Waterloo.

Medora, N., J. Larson, N. Hortacsu, and D. Parul. 2002. "Perceived Attitudes Toward Romanticism." *Journal of Comparative Family Studies* 33:155–78.

Meier, B. 2005. "Using Metaphor to Promote Happiness: Will Directing People to Attend Up Make Them 'Feel Up'?" Ph.D. dissertation, North Dakota State University.

Melnarik, C. 1999. "Retaining High Tech Employees." Ph.D. dissertation, Walden University.

Memory Clinic. 2002. "Ginkgo Fails to Aid Memory in Double-Blind Study."

Mendoza, J. C. 1999. "Resiliency Factors in High School Students at Risk for Academic Failure." Ph.D. dissertation, California School of Professional Psychology.

Meulemann, H. 2001. "Life Satisfaction from Late Adolescence to Mid-Life." *Journal of Happiness Studies* 2 (4): 445–65.

Michalos, A. 2005. "Arts and the Quality of Life: An Exploratory Study." *Social Indicators Research* 71:11–59

Miner, A., T. Glomb, and C. Hulin. 2005. "Experience Sampling Mood and Its Correlates at Work." *Journal of Occupational and Organizational Psychology* 78:171–93.

Moeller, J., and O. Koeller. 2000. "Spontaneous and Reactive Attributions Following Academic Achievement." *Social Psychology of Education* 4:67–86.

Morman, M., and K. Floyd. 2002. "A 'changing culture of fatherhood': Effects on Affectionate Communication, Closeness, and Satisfaction in Men's Relationships with Their Fathers and Their Sons." *Western Journal of Communication* 66 (4): 395–411.

Mount Sinai School of Medicine. 2003. "Teens and Tanning: A Dangerous Combination."

Murray, S., and J. Holmes. 1999. "The Mental Ties That Bind: Cognitive Structures That Predict Relationship Resilience." *Journal of Personality and Social Psychology* 77:1228–44.

Murray, S., J. Holmes, and D. Griffin. 2000. "Self-Esteem and the Quest for Felt Security: How Perceived Regard Regulates Attachment Processes." *Journal of Personality and Social Psychology* 78:478–98.

Nair, E. 2000. "Health and Aging." *Journal of Adult Development* 7 (2): 121–26.

Nanayakkara, A. 2002. "A Cultural Perspective on the Role of Self-Determination in Personal Relationships." Ph.D. dissertation, University of Houston.

National Cancer Institute. 2002. "Many Young Americans Risk Skin Cancer from Annual Sunburns."

National Sleep Foundation. 2003. "Poor Sleep Linked to Earlier Death in Older Adults."

Natural Resources Defense Council. 2002. "What's in Bottled Water?"

Nock, S. 2001. "The Marriages of Equally Dependent Spouses." *Journal of Family Issues* 22:755–75.

North Dakota State University. 1999. "Journal Writing Can Alleviate Illnesses."

O'Brien, V., M. Martinez-Pons, and M. Kopala. 1999. "Mathematics Self-Efficacy, Ethnic Identity, Gender, and Career Interests Related to Mathematics and Science." *Journal of Educational Research* 92:231–35.

Ohio State University. 2002. "One-On-One with Pharmacists Gives Patients Medication Advantage."

Oregon Department of Human Services. 2002. "Piercing Your Ears? Stick to the Lobes."

Orlick, T. 1998. *Embracing Your Potential.* Champaign, IL: Human Kinetics.

Othaganont, P., C. Sinthuvorakan, and P. Jensupakarn. 2002. "Daily Living Practice of the Life-Satisfied Thai Elderly." *Journal of Transcultural Nursing* 13 (1): 24–29.

Oxford University. 2002a. "Calming Women in Labor with Aromatherapy."

———. 2002b. "Inefficacy of Reducing Number of Meals."

Pallen, R. 2001. "Intimacy, Need Fulfillment, and Violence in Marital Relationships." Ph.D. dissertation, University of Arkansas.

Palmer-Daley, J. 2001. "Imagination: The Stuff That Love Is Made Of." Ph.D. dissertation, Pacifica Graduate Institute.

Pape, A. 2001. "Conflict Resolution Satisfaction: A Study of Satisfied Marriages Across 16 Domains of Marital Conflict." Ph.D. dissertation, Texas Women's University.

Paris, J. 1999. "Identity Consolidation in Early Adulthood: Relations with Ego-Resiliency, the Context of Marriage, and Personality Changes." *Journal of Personality* 67:295–329.

Pauk, W. 1997. *How to Study in College.* Boston: Houghton Mifflin.

Peiperl, M., and Y. Baruch. 1997. "Back to Square Zero: The Post Corporate Career." *Organizational Dynamics* 25:7–22.

Pennsylvania State University. 2002a. "Holidays and Stress-Eating."

———. 2002b. "Sense of Control Eases Physical Toll of Stressful Situation."

———. 2002c. "Super-Hydration."

Persley, R. 1998. "Towards a New Understanding of Organizational Behavior, Sport, and Peak Performance Phenomena." Ph.D. dissertation, Union Institute.

Peters, B., J. Joireman, and R. Ridgway. 2005. "Individual Differences in the Consideration of Future Consequences Scale Correlate with Sleep Habits, Sleep Quality, and GPA in University Students." *Psychological Reports* 96:817–24.

Peterson, R., M. Cannito, and S. Brown. 1995. "An Exploratory Investigation of Voice Characteristics and Selling Effectiveness." *Journal of Personal Selling and Sales Management* 15:1–15.

Philpot, C. 2001. "Someday My Prince Will Come." In *Casebook for Integrating Family Therapy,* ed. S. McDaniel and D. Lusterman. Washington, DC: American Psychological Association.

Polivy, J., and C. P. Herman. 1999. "The Effects of Resolving to Diet on Restrained and Unrestrained Eaters." *International Journal of Eating Disorders* 26:434–47.

———. 2000. "The False-Hope Syndrome: Unfulfilled Expectations of Self-Change." *Current Directions in Psychological Science* 9:128–31.

Pollock, K. 1998. "The Relationship Between Leadership Style and Subordinate Satisfaction and Performance in Public Accounting Firms." Ph.D. dissertation, University of Kentucky.

Porter, G. 2001. "Workaholics as High-Performance Employees: The Intersection of Workplace and Family Relationship Problems." In *High-Performing Families:*

Causes, Consequences, and Clinical Solutions, ed. B. Robinson, and N. Chase. Washington, DC: American Counseling Association.

Prescott, C., and K. Kendler. 2001. "Associations Between Marital Status and Alcohol Consumption in a Longitudinal Study of Female Twins." *Journal of Studies on Alcohol* 62:589–604.

Protinsky, H., and L. Coward. 2001. "Developmental Lessons of Seasoned Marital and Family Therapists: A Qualitative Investigation." *Journal of Marital and Family Therapy* 27:375–84.

Ramanaiah, N., and F. Detwiler. 1997. "Life Satisfaction and the Five-Factor Model of Personality." *Psychological Reports* 80:1208.

Reboussin, B., W. J. Rejeski, K. Martin, and K. Callahan. 2000. "Correlates of Satisfaction with Body Function and Body Appearance in Middle- and Older Aged Adults." *Psychology and Health* 15 (2): 239–54.

Ricaurte, R. A. 1999. "Student Success in a Communicative Classroom: A Grounded Theory." Ph.D. dissertation, University of Nebraska.

Richburg, M. 1998. "The Relationship Between Dyadic Adjustment and the Structure, Satisfaction, and Intimacy of Married Men's Same-Sex Friendships." Ph.D. dissertation, University of Denver.

Roberts, N., and R. Levenson. 2001. "The Remains of the Workday: Impact of Job Stress and Exhaustion on Marital Interaction in Police Couples." *Journal of Marriage and the Family* 63:1052–67.

Robeson, R. 1998. "College Students on the Rebound." Ph.D. dissertation, Indiana University.

Robinson-Rowe, M. 2002. "Meaning and Satisfaction in the Lives of Midlife, Never-Married Heterosexual Women." Ph.D. dissertation, Alliant International University.

Rogers, S., and D. DeBoer. 2001. "Changes in Wives' Income: Effects on Marital Happiness, Psychological Well-Being, and the Risk of Divorce." *Journal of Marriage and the Family* 63:458–72.

Roloff, M., K. Soule, and C. Carey. 2001. "Reasons for Remaining in a Relationship and Responses to Relational Transgressions." *Journal of Social and Personal Relationships* 18:362–85.

Romero-Medina, A. 2001. "Sex Equal Stable Marriages." *Theory and Decision* 50:197–212.

Ruef, A. 2001. "Empathy in Long-Term Marriage: Behavioral and Physiological Correlates." Ph.D. dissertation, University of California, Berkeley.

Rundle-Gardiner, A., and S. Carr. 2005. "Quitting a Workplace That Discourages Achievement Motivation: Do Individual Differences Matter?" *New Zealand Journal of Psychology* 34:149–56.

Russell, M., and M. Atwater. 2005. "Traveling the Road to Success: A Discourse on Persistence Throughout the Science Pipeline with African American Students at a Predominantly White Institution." *Journal of Research in Science Teaching* 42:691–715.

Ryan, L., and S. Dziurawiec. 2001. "Materialism and Its Relationship to Life Satisfaction." *Social Indicators Research* 55 (2): 185–97.

Saitama Medical School. 2003. "Effects of Air Travel on Circulation."

Sarkisian, C., R. Hays, S. Berry, and C. Mangione. 2001. "Expectations Regarding Aging Among Older Adults and Physicians Who Care for Older Adults." *Medical Care* 39 (9): 1025–36.

Scherneck, M. 1998. "The Relationship Between Self-Esteem and Academic Performance." Ph.D. dissertation, State University of New York at Albany.

Schminke, M., M. Ambrose, and D. Neubaum. 2005. "The Effect of Leader Moral Development on Ethical Climate and Employee Attitudes." *Organizational Behavior and Human Decision Processes* 97:135–51.

Schneewind, K., and A. Gerhard. 2002. "Relationship Personality, Conflict Resolution, and Marital Satisfaction in the First 5 Years of Marriage." *Family Relations* 51:63–71.

Schulman, P. 1999. "Applying Learned Optimism to Increase Sales Productivity." *Journal of Personal Selling and Sales Management* 19:31–37.

Schwartz, R. 2000. *Marriage in Motion: The Natural Ebb and Flow of Lasting Relationships.* Cambridge, MA: Perseus Publishing.

Sedlacek, W. 1999. "Black Students on White Campuses." *Journal of College Student Development* 40:538–50.

Shank, M., and F. Beasley. 1998. "Fan or Fanatic: Refining a Measure of Sports Involvement." *Journal of Sport Behavior* 21:435

Sigmund, E. 1999. "Consciously Directing the Creative Process in Business." *Transactional Analysis Journal* 29:222–27.

Silverman, L. 1998. "Through the Lens of Giftedness." *Roeper Review* 20:204–10.

Simons, C. 2002. "Proactive Coping, Perceived Self-Efficacy, and Locus of Control as Predictors of Life Satisfaction in Young, Middle-Aged, and Older Adults." Ph.D. dissertation, Georgia State University.

Smith, A. 2000. "Understanding the Impact of the Founder's Legacy in Current Organizational Behavior." In *Dynamic Consultation in a Changing Workplace,* ed. E. Klein. Madison, CT: Psychosocial Press.

Sparkes, A. 1998. "Athletic Identity: An Achilles' Heel to the Survival of Self." *Qualitative Health Research* 8:644–64.

Sparrow, K. R. 1998. "Resiliency and Vulnerability in Girls During Cognitively Challenging Tasks." Ph.D. dissertation, Florida State University, Tallahassee.

Sprecher, S., and D. Felmlee. 2000. "Romantic Partners' Perceptions of Social Network Attributes with the Passage of Time and Relationship Transitions." *Personal Relationships* 7:325–40.

Stanford University. 2002a. "Air Pollution Linked to Increased Medical Care and Costs for Elderly."

———. 2002b. "Sex Discrimination in Your Medicine Cabinet."

———. 2003. "Link Between Grape Juice Consumption and Lowered Risk of Heart Trouble."

State University of New York at Buffalo. 2003a. "Health Benefits of Moderate Drinking May Not Apply to African-Americans."

———. 2003b. "Pets in the Home Lower Blood Pressure."

Steger, M., P. Frazier, S. Oishi, and M. Kaler. 2006. "The Meaning in Life Questionnaire: Assessing the Presence of and Search for Meaning in Life." *Journal of Counseling Psychology* 53:80–93.

Sternberg, R., G. Forsythe, J. Hedlund, J. Horvath, R. Wagner, W. Williams, S. Snook, and E. Grigorenko. 2000. *Practical Intelligence in Everyday Life.* New York: Cambridge University Press.

Stewart, G., K. Carson, and R. Cardy. 1996. "The Joint Effects of Conscientiousness and Self-Leadership Training on Employee Self-Directed Behavior in a Service Setting." *Personnel Psychology* 49:143–64.

Sullivan, K. 2001. "Understanding the Relationship Between Religiosity and Marriage: An Investigation of the Immediate and Longitudinal Effects of Religiosity on Newlywed Couples." *Journal of Family Psychology* 15:610–26.

Sumer, H. C., and P. Knight. 2001. "How Do People with Different Attachment Styles Balance Work and Family? A Personality Perspective on Work-Family Linkage." *Journal of Applied Psychology* 86:653–63.

Sweeney, M. 2002. "Remarriage and the Nature of Divorce: Does It Matter Which Spouse Chose to Leave?" *Journal of Family Issues* 23:410–40.

Symmonds-Mueth, J. 2000. "Adult Males: Marital Satisfaction and General Life Contentment Across the Life Cycle." Ph.D. dissertation, University of Missouri, St. Louis.

Szinovacz, M., and S. DeViney. 1999. "The Retiree Identity." *Journal of Gerontology* 54:207–18.

Szinovacz, M., and A. Schaffer. 2000. "Effects of Retirement on Marital Conflict Tactics." *Journal of Family Issues* 21:367–89.

Tamir, M. 2005. "Don't Worry, Be Happy? Neuroticism, Trait-Consistent Affect Regulation, and Performance." *Journal of Personality and Social Psychology* 89:449–61.

Taylor, D. 2001. "Weaving Modern-Day Wives' Tales: Women Redefining Wifehood." Ph.D. dissertation, Texas Tech University.

Thomas, J. 1999. "Relationship Efficacy: The Prediction of Goal Attainment by Dating Couples." Ph.D. dissertation, University of Maryland.

Thornton, A., and L. Young-DeMarco. 2001. "Four Decades of Trends in Attitudes Toward Family Issues in the United States." *Journal of Marriage and the Family* 63:1009–37.

Thornton, F., G. Privette, and C. Bundrick. 1999. "Peak Performance of Business Leaders: An Experience Parallel to Self-Actualization Theory." *Journal of Business and Psychology* 14:253–64.

Tokyo Metropolitan Consumer Center. 2002. "Ameliorating Unhealthy Air in Households."

Toth, J., R. Brown, and X. Xu. 2002. "Separate Family and Community Realities? An Urban-Rural Comparison of the Association Between Family Life Satisfaction and Community Satisfaction." *Community, Work and Family* 5:181–202.

Tufts University. 2003. "Checklist of Claims May Signal Trouble on Internet Cancer-Treatment Sites."

Tulane University. 2002. "Foods Rich in Folate May Reduce Risk of Stroke."

Tuuli, P., and S. Karisalmi. 1999. "Impact of Working Life Quality on Burnout." *Experimental Aging Research* 25:441–49.

U.S. Department of Health and Human Services. 2002. "Ideal Body Images."

University Hospital, Innsbruck, Austria. 2002. "Fertility and the Mountain Biker."

University of Arkansas. 2002. "Memory Isn't Lost—Just Out of Sync."

University of Alabama at Birmingham. 2002. "Half of Heart Attack Patients Drive to Hospital."

University of Bradford. 1999. "Effects of Absolutist Thinking."

University of California, Irvine. 2002. "Teen Anxiety, Chances of Harmful Smoking and Eating Behavior Higher Than Expected."

University of California, Los Angeles. 2002. "Home Life Effects Health."

University of Chicago. 2002. "Lonely People Face Higher Risk of Heart Disease."

University of Hull. 2002. "Guilt and the Immune System."

University of Illinois. 2002. "Effects of Walking Regimen Tested."

University of Illinois at Chicago. 2003. "Exposing Anti-Aging Propaganda."

University of Iowa. 2002a. "Common Painkiller May Hinder Aspirin's Effects."

———. 2002b. "Connection Between Personality, Death Among Chronically Ill."

———. 2002c. "Little 'Weekend Effect' Related to Intensive Care Admissions."

University of Kentucky. 2002. "Fear of the Unlikely."

University of Maryland. 2002. "Can Forgiveness Make the Immune System Stronger?"

University of Maryland Baltimore County. 2002. "Salutary Effects of Laughter on Long-Term Health."

University of Michigan. 2002a. "100 Million Americans Live with Aching Backs."

———. 2002b. "Effects of Temporary Stress."

———. 2002c. "Household Hazards."

University of Minnesota. 2002a. "Supportive Spouse, Family, Friends Contribute to 'Successful Aging.'"

———. 2002b. "Building Stamina over Time."

University of Missouri. 2002. "Alleviating Stress Effects in Men."

University of North Carolina. 2002a. "Home Injury Found to Be a Major Cause of Deaths."

———. 2002b. "Nearness of Supermarkets Boosts People's Intake of Nutritious Fruits, Vegetables."

———. 2003. "Effects of Contact on Stress."

University of Pittsburgh. 2002. "Varied Implications of Periodontal Disease."

University of Richmond. 2002. "Fitness Can Be Free."

University of Southern California. 2002. "Whitening May Cause Short-Term Tooth Sensitivity."

University of Texas. 2002. "Caffeine-Signaling Activity in Brain Function."

University of Texas Southwestern Medical Center. 2002a. "Time to Debunk Cold-Season Myths."

———. 2002b. "Use Caution, Ask Questions Before Attending Botox Party."

University of Toronto. 2002a. "Driving Dangers Vary by Day and Time."

———. 2002b. "Work and Marriage Influences Blood Pressure."

University of Virginia. 2002. "Unintended Effects of Blowing Your Nose."

University of Washington. 2003. "Age Affects Taste of Vegetables."

University of Wisconsin. 2003. "Meditation Effects on Immune System."

Van Boven, L. 2005. "Experientialism, Materialism, and the Pursuit of Happiness." *Review of General Psychology* 9:132–42.

Van Handel Eagles, J. 1999. "An Inquiry into the Incidence and Nature of Mentoring Relationships in Women over the Age of Sixty." Ph.D. dissertation, Walden University.

Van Willigen, M. 2000. "Differential Benefits of Volunteering Across the Life Course." *Journals of Gerontology: Psychological Sciences and Social Sciences* 55 (5): 308–18.

Vaughn, L. 2001. "The Relationship Between Marital Satisfaction Levels Associated with Participation in the Free and Hope-Focused Marital Enrichment Program." Ph.D. dissertation, Regent University.

Veenhoven, R. 2005. "Is Life Getting Better?: How Long and Happily Do People Live in Modern Society?" *European Psychologist* 10:330–43.

Velting, D. 1999. "Personality and Negative Expectations: Trait Structure of the Beck Hopelessness Scale." *Personality and Individual Differences* 26:913–21.

Verbeke, W., and R. Bagozzi. 2000. "Sales Call Anxiety: Exploring What It Means When Fear Rules a Sales Encounter." *Journal of Marketing* 64:88–101.

Vinograde, D. 2001. "Black and White Heterosexual Women's Marital and Same-Sex Best Friend Relationships, and the Contributions of Entitlement, Relationship Equality and Relationship Intimacy to Well-Being." Ph.D. dissertation, Adelphi University.

Visher, E., J. Visher, and K. Pasley. 2003. "Remarriage Families and Stepparenting." In *Normal Family Processes: Growing Diversity and Complexity,* ed. F. Walsh. New York: Guilford Press.

Wallace, K., T. Bisconti, and C. Bergeman. 2001. "The Mediational Effect of Hardiness on Social Support and Optimal Outcomes in Later Life." *Basic and Applied Social Psychology* 23 (4): 267–79.

Walther-Lee, D. 1999. "The Changing Role of Grandparents: Adult Children's Memories of Their Grandparents." Ph.D. dissertation, Adelphi University.

Ward, M. 2002. "Does Television Exposure Affect Emerging Adults' Attitudes and Assumptions About Sexual Relationships?" *Journal of Youth and Adolescence* 31:1–15.

Waschull, S. 2005. "Predicting Success in Online Psychology Courses: Self-Discipline and Motivation." *Teaching of Psychology* 32:190–92.

Watson, D., B. Hubbard, and D. Wiese. 2000a. "General Traits of Personality and Affectivity as Predictors of Satisfaction in Intimate Relationships: Evidence from Self and Partner Ratings." *Journal of Personality* 68:413–49.

———. 2000b. "Self-Other Agreement in Personality and Affectivity: The Role of Acquaintanceship, Trait Visibility, and Assumed Similarity." *Journal of Personality and Social Psychology* 78:465–558.

Weigel, D., and D. Ballard-Reisch. 1999. "All Marriages Are Not Maintained Equally: Marital Type, Marital Quality, and the Use of Maintenance Behaviors." *Personal Relationships* 6 (3): 291–303.

Werneck De Almeida, E. S. 1999. "Social Integration and Academic Confidence." Ph.D. dissertation, University of Hartford.

Werner, E., and R. Smith. 2001. *Journeys from Childhood to Midlife: Risk, Resilience, and Recovery.* Ithaca, NY: Cornell University Press.

Whatley, A. 1998. "Gifted Women and Teaching: A Compatible Choice?" *Roeper Review* 21:117–24.

Wiese, B., and A. Freund. 2005. "Goal Progress Makes One Happy, or Does It? Longitudinal Findings from the Work Domain." *Journal of Occupational and Organizational Psychology* 78:287–304.

Wiesenfeld, B., S. Raghuram, and G. Raghu. 1999. "Managers in a Virtual Context." In *Trends in Organizational Behavior,* ed. C. Cooper. New York: Wiley and Sons.

Williams, A., D. Haber, G. Weaver, and J. Freeman. 1998. "Altruistic Activity." *Activities, Adaptation, and Aging* 22:31.

Williams, E., E. Soeprapto, K. Like, P. Touradji, S. Hess, and C. Hill. 1998. "Perceptions of Serendipity." *Journal of Counseling Psychology* 45:379–89.

Winslow, L., 2001. "The Relationship of Gambling on Depression, Perceived Social Support, and Life Satisfaction in an Elderly Sample." Ph.D. dissertation, Hofstra University.

World Health Organization. 2001. "Sick-Building Syndrome."

Wu, P. 1998. "Goal Structures of Materialists vs. Non-Materialists." Ph.D. dissertation, University of Michigan.

———. 2001. "Analysis of the Effects of Marriage Encounter as a Form of Family Life Education." Ph.D. dissertation, Claremont Graduate University.

Yamada, N. 2000. "The Relationship Between Leisure Activities, Psycho-Social Development and Life Satisfaction in Late Adulthood." *Japanese Journal of Developmental Psychology* 11 (1): 34–44.

Zeidner, M., and E. J. Schleyer. 1999. "The Big Fish Little Pond Effect for Academic Self-Concept, Test Anxiety, and School Grades in Gifted Children." *Contemporary Educational Psychology* 24:305–29.

Zhou, J., and J. George. 2001. "When Job Dissatisfaction Leads to Creativity: Encouraging the Expression of Voice." *Academy of Management Journal* 44 (4): 682–96.

Zink, D. 2000. "The Enduring Marriages of Adult Children of Divorce." Ph.D. dissertation, St. Louis University.

Acknowledgments

I offer my appreciation to Gideon Weil and the staff at HarperSan-Francisco, and to my agent, Sandy Choron. Without their continuing efforts, this book would not exist. My great thanks to TinaGayle Niven for her help in the final tasks of taking the hundreds of pages on my office floor and bringing them to you.

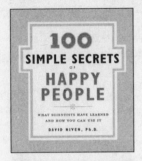
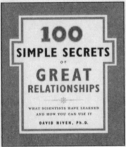
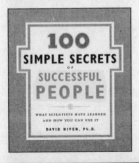
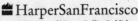